How to Prevent and Heal
RUNNING
and Other Sports
INJURIES

Also by ERIC GOLANTY:

Human Reproduction

How to Prevent and Heal RUNNING and Other Sports INJURIES

Eric Golanty, M.A., M.S.

Illustrations by David Wellner

South Brunswick and New York: A. S. Barnes and Company
London: Thomas Yoseloff Ltd

A. S. Barnes and Co., Inc.
Cranbury, New Jersey 08512

Thomas Yoseloff Ltd
Magdalen House
136-148 Tooley Street
London SE1 2TT, England

Library of Congress Cataloging in Publication Data

Golanty, Eric.
  How to prevent running and other sports injuries

  Bibliography: p.
  Includes index.
  1. Running—Accident and injuries—Prevention.
2. Sports—Accidents and injuries—Prevention.
3. Sports medicine. I. Title.
RC1220.R8G64   617'.1027   78-75305
ISBN 0-498-02391-5 (cloth)
ISBN 0-498-02480-6 (paperback)

Printed in the United States of America

Contents

Acknowledgments   7
Introduction   9

Part 1: Understanding Sports Injuries

1   How the Body Moves   15
2   Dealing with Sports Injuries   21
3   Types of Common Sports Injuries   27

Part 2: Preventing Sports Injuries

4   Be in Shape   35
5   Improve Flexibility and Form   42
6   Strengthen Muscles   52
7   Use Good Equipment   72

Part 3: Specific Sports Injuries

8   Foot and Ankle Problems   81
9   Leg Problems   86
10 Knee Problems   94
11 Hip, Back, and Pelvic Problems   100

12   Shoulder, Arm, and Hand Problems   107
13   Skin Problems   112
14   Injuries in Various Sports   117
Bibliography   132
Index   133

Acknowledgments

My special thanks to Dr. Bernie Feldman, Molly Shinn, and John Stanovich for helping me to make this book happen.

Introduction

It is estimated that there are over 70 million amateur athletes in the United States taking part in numerous sports—tennis, jogging, swimming, weekend touch football, softball, cycling, golf, bowling, skiing, and volleyball, just to name a few. And although these millions of people are participating in different sports, they nevertheless face a common problem: the sports injury.

I decided to write this book when I once became sidelined from my usual running routine. It was during that idle and sometimes painful two-month period that I came to realize how many of my athletically active friends suffered their own versions of my knee ailment. Each one seemed to have a "complaint of the week," some ache or stiffness or skin problem that was causing trouble. Yet rarely did any of us have a clear idea of what ailed us. Because these injuries were rarely incapacitating, few of us went to the doctor. Whether it was a bout with sore knees, blistered feet, pulled muscles, or tennis elbow, we would simply hang in there until the pain went away and we could become active again.

I soon realized that what I needed, and what a lot of amateur athletes needed, was a book that explained sports injuries and how to avoid some of them. College and professional athletes have the expert advice of trainers and team physicians to help them with their sports-related ailments, but the amateur very often has to fend for him or herself.

Being a college health teacher, science writer, and lifelong jock who has had his share of sports injuries, I was able to put together this guide to understanding and avoiding sports injuries by gathering information from the literature in sports medicine and by consulting athletes, trainers, and coaches.

Sports injuries usually occur in the musculoskeletal system of the body—the muscles, bones, ligaments, tendons, and joints. There are thousands of scientific terms and concepts that describe this system and the traumas to it. I have tried to limit the length of this book and still provide a reasonably thorough account of how the system works and what goes wrong to cause an injury.

I hope my efforts will be of some help to you.

A Word to the Wise

This book is not intended to replace competent medical care. If you become injured in your sport, you will have to decide whether or not to seek professional treatment. Certainly if the injury causes a lot of pain or loss of function, then you should probably see a specialist. Try to find someone who specializes in sports injuries—not because the treatment necessarily will be better, but because that specialist will likely understand the need of the athletically inclined to return to sports activity as soon as possible and can perhaps gear treatment to fulfill that desire.

Eric Golanty

How to Prevent and Heal
RUNNING
and Other Sports
INJURIES

Part 1

Understanding Sports Injuries

1 How the Body Moves

Many amateur athletes know very little about how their bodies actually work. If you are one of the lucky ones who never experience aches, pains, bruises, pulled muscles, stiffness, and temporary disability from athletic injuries, then it probably doesn't matter if you are also ignorant of the basics of body movement. But if you are like the rest of us, constantly doing battle with some sort of pain or other, then a rudimentary understanding of the body's primary movement system—the muscles, bones, ligaments, tendons, and joints—can probably help you take care of your minor sports injuries, better understand the treatment you may receive from a medical specialist, and prevent future injuries.

The Movement System

Basically, any body movement, whether it involves bending, turning, jumping, or grasping, is the result of bones being moved when a muscle or group of muscles contracts.

Muscles are made up of bands of protein fibers that have the ability to shorten or contract. In the contraction process, the fibers slide past each other to shorten the muscle. Shortening is all that muscles can do; that is how they work. Movement occurs because muscles are attached to bones. When muscles contract they exert a pulling force on a bone and cause it to move. The greater the number of muscle fibers, the greater the pulling force on the bone.

Muscles are attached to bones by tough fibrous bands called *tendons*. Unlike muscles, tendons are not contractile tissues, although they are capable of some stretching. The sole function of tendon is to attach muscle to bone. Usually the junction of a tendon and muscle is an interwoven network of tendon and muscle fibers; therefore, a muscle and its tendon are often considered as one functional unit.

As an example of the action of one part of the primary movement system, consider the bending of the arm at the elbow.

Hold your arm out straight and then bend it, bringing your hand to your shoulder. This movement is called *elbow* or *forearm flexion*. (Whenever a movement decreases the angle between two bones, it is called flexion.) Put your other hand on the top part of the arm you have flexed, on the *biceps* muscle, and flex a few more times. The biceps muscle is the one that little kids show off when they "make a muscle."

As you bend your arm, you will feel the biceps bulge every time you flex. This occurs because the biceps is contracting when you move your forearm. Actually, there are two other muscles in the upper arm that are involved in elbow flexion, but they are not as easy to feel. All three muscles tend to act as a group and are often referred to as the *forearm* or *elbow flexors*.

The elbow is an example of a joint. Anatomically speaking, a joint is a skeletal structure where two or more bones meet or *articulate*.

Many body movements occur at joints. In fact, nearly all fluid movements are possible because of joints. Without them we would walk around stiff and straight. Joints allow us to bend and rotate parts of the skeleton relative to each other.

The bones in a joint are held together by tough fibrous structures called *ligaments*. Not only do ligaments hold bones together, but they also provide support to prevent the bones from coming apart *(dislocating)* when an unusually severe stress is placed on a joint. Muscles and tendons also provide support for joints.

Three bones make up the elbow joint. They include the large bone

16

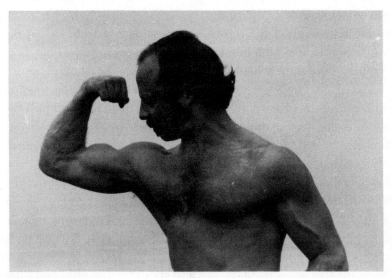

Howard's biceps.

of the upper arm called the *humerus* and two bones of the forearm, the *radius,* on the thumb side of the forearm, and the *ulna,* on the little-finger side of the forearm. Several ligaments attach the humerus to the radius and the ulna, and there is a ligamentous attachment between the radius and ulna as well.

Therefore, when you flex your arm what you are doing is pulling the radius and ulna closer to the humerus. The biceps and other elbow flexors originate on the upper part of the humerus and also in part of the shoulder, and extend across the elbow joint to the two forearm bones. When the muscles contract, they pull the forearm bones toward the humerus.

The elbow joint, like all other moveable joints, has a lubricating system to allow freer movement. One part of the lubricating system is *cartilage,* an elastic material that covers the ends of the articulating surfaces of the bones. The cartilage helps prevent the wearing away by friction of the ends of the bones as they move against each other.

Another part of the joint lubricating system is a membrane that surrounds the entire joint. The membrane is attached to the bones of the joint and completely encapsulates the junction of the bones. The inside part of the membrane, called the *synovial membrane,* makes a lubricating fluid called *synovial fluid,* which has a consistency similar to egg white.

On the back side of the upper arm there is a muscle called the *triceps,* which is also attached to the humerus and the two bones of the forearm. When the triceps contracts, it pulls the forearm toward the back of the upper arm, and if it were not for the special construction of the elbow joint, the triceps, in theory, could pull the forearm all the way in the opposite direction. Instead, the triceps pulls the arm straight (actually, a little more than 180 degrees), which is called *extension.*

It is possible to think of movements at most joints in terms of the actions of flexor muscles, which bend the joint, and extensor muscles, which straighten it. There are flexor and extensor muscle groups of the wrist, elbow, hip, shoulder, knee, ankle, fingers, and, toes.

There are also muscles in the hip and shoulder that effect rotation at these joints. And there are muscles that pull a body part like an arm, leg, or finger away from the body midline. These are called *abductors.* The muscles that oppose the action of these muscles are called *adductors.* The action of any group of muscles is always opposed by another group called the *antagonists.*

The Brain and Movement

Muscles, bones, ligaments, tendons, and joints are not the only components of the body's primary movement system, although that is where most sports injuries tend to occur. The brain and peripheral nerves are also parts of the system.

Every voluntary (as opposed to reflexive) movement begins as a command from the brain that is sent to the muscles through the nerve network of the body. When a muscle receives nervous stimulation, it contracts, causing the bone to which it is attached to move.

When you move any part of your body, you do not consciously decide what every muscle in the movement should do and then proceed to contract and relax those muscles individually. Instead, you decide what you want to do and your brain automatically coordinates all the appropriate body parts to effect your wish.

18

Most coordinated movement is controlled by a region on the surface of the brain called the *motor cortex*. Actually, there are two motor corteces, one on each cerebral hemisphere. The right motor cortex controls movement on the left side of the body, and the left motor cortex controls movement on the right.

We know about the motor cortex from some remarkable experiments that were carried out by neurosurgeons during brain operations, usually for the treatment of epilepsy or brain tumors. These experiments showed that when a part of the cortex, now known to be the motor cortex, was stimulated by a tiny electric current, some part of the body would move completely without the patient's volition. By touching several areas it was possible to map the motor cortex to

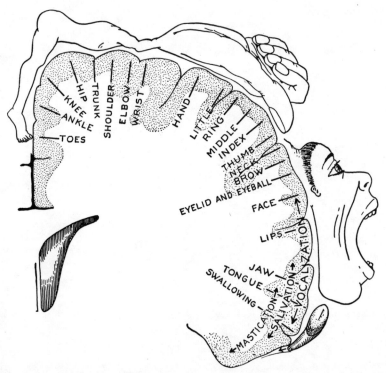

The motor homunculus. **Reproduced with permission from Penfield and Rasmussen, *The Cerebral Cortex of Man.* Macmillan, 1950.**

19

determine which brain regions control movement in which parts of the body.

An incredibly bizarre picture has been concocted to illustrate what is called the *motor homunculus*. It is a disjointed body displayed over the cortex to show the body region controlled by that part of the cortex. There's absolutely no correlation between actual body anatomy and the anatomy as displayed on the motor cortex. Moreover, there is no correlation between the size of the brain area and the size of the body area it controls. The regions of the body that have the greatest representation on the motor cortex are the hand and the mouth. This is because these regions require the most muscle control to execute the fine movements necessary for dexterity and speech.

2 Dealing with Sports Injuries

It is hard to find someone who is athletically active who has not also had to deal with a sports-related injury. Just about everyone has been hurt in sports in one way or another: jamming a finger in a friendly volleyball game; colliding with a handball opponent and bruising an arm or a leg; twisting an ankle by stepping in a sprinkler hole in the park while jogging or chasing a fly ball.

Regardless of the type of injury and how it happened, there are things a person can do to deal with a sports injury to facilitate healing and regain activity. This is true whether or not medical help is sought. Two of the most important are the application of specific first-aid measures as soon as possible and the engaging in a conscientious rehabilitation program to strengthen the injured region and thereby prevent future injury.

Inflammation and Repair

The physiological response to most injuries is the same regardless of the type of damage and the region of the body that is involved. The response is characterized by this sequence of events:

1. Substances from the damaged tissues promote the accumulation of fluid in the injured region.

2. Local internal bleeding occurs but eventually stops, and a fibrous clot, called a *hematoma,* forms.
3. White blood cells accumulate in the injured region to clear away tissue debris and foreign material such as bacteria.

This response is called *inflammation,* and it is characterized by local swelling, redness, sometimes loss of function, and pain. Pain is caused by fluid and other substances released from the damaged tissue stimulating certain nerve fibers that cause the sensation of pain. Pain is important for it tells us something is wrong and usually stops us from continuing whatever we were doing and making the injury worse.

When the inflammation has subsided, which usually takes a few days (unless the injured region continues to receive stress), repair and healing can take place. This process is mediated by special cells called *fibroblasts,* which invade the damaged region and secrete fibrous material that knits torn or broken pieces of muscle, tendon, or ligament together. The repair of a muscle can take several days and even in the worst tears the healing is complete in a couple of weeks. Tendons and ligaments are repaired more slowly, however. The blood supply to these tissues is normally not substantial, and therefore nutrients needed for the repair gather slowly. Tendons and ligaments may need up to eight weeks to heal.

First Aid for Injuries

If you are playing tennis and you or someone else on the court severely twists an ankle or pulls a thigh muscle, what can be done immediately to help?

Because these and nearly all sports injuries involve the inflammation response, a helpful immediate treatment is to limit the swelling and internal blood loss as much as possible. Not only will this diminish the fluid accumulation in the injured area, but it will also lessen the pain and promote healing.

How do you administer this miraculous treatment? With I.C.E.—an acronym used by trainers, coaches, and sports physicians for "*I*ce, *C*ompression, and *E*levation." For twenty-four to seventy-two hours after an injury, depending on its extent, the

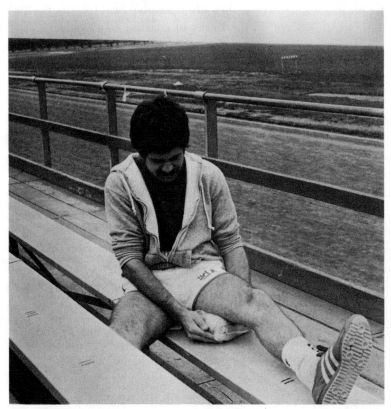

Icing a pulled hamstring.

injured region should get frequent ice treatments, generally three times a day, be wrapped in an elastic bandage, and elevated. To ice an injury simply fill a plastic grocery bag with crushed ice or ice cubes, and put it directly on the injured area. Some people might find it easier to put an entire forearm or foot in a bucket of ice water. Apply the ice for five to ten minutes each time.

The cold causes blood vessels to constrict and prevents additional fluid from entering the injured area. This fluid causes swelling and stimulates pain fibers.

When the swelling and internal bleeding have stopped, you can then apply therapeutic measures to promote healing. Although these vary depending on the injury, they often involve heat treatments and stretching exercises within the limits of comfort.

In addition, it may be wise to immobilize a region until the damaged tissues heal. This prevents continued internal bleeding, allows blood clots to clear up, and gives the fibers of muscles, tendons, and ligaments the opportunity to knit properly. Because the repair of tendons and ligaments may take weeks, the injured region may benefit from being kept relatively immobile (either bandaged, in a sling, or in a plaster or fiberglass cast) to give the repair processes the opportunity to take place without disturbance.

Fortunately, most sports injuries involve bumps, twists, and tears that may be painful but not usually life threatening. However, if someone has been hurt and is unconscious, is bleeding profusely, or has stopped breathing, then a first-class medical emergency exists. Cover the injured person with a blanket or jacket, and call an ambulance, a fire department paramedic unit, or a doctor. Those who know CPR (cardiopulmonary resuscitation) or have Red Cross training in first aid may administer help until the professionals arrive. And contrary to what is sometimes seen in the movies, seriously hurt people should not receive alcohol to revive them. Alcohol is a nervous system depressant and may impair breathing and the body's own attempts to overcome the injury.

If a bone has been broken and is protruding through the skin or there is an obvious deformation of part of the skeleton, do not move the injured person. You may make matters worse by causing internal injury. Try not to move the person even if you are out in the country and far from a phone. It would be better if someone stayed with the injured person and someone else went for help. Whatever the situation, use your common sense.

Serious bleeding should be stopped immediately. To stop blood loss, apply pressure with a pressure bandage on the open wound. The object is to keep the blood inside. Direct pressure is preferable to the use of a tourniquet, which can cut off blood to the entire region and may lead to damage of all the internal structures near the wound.

Rehabilitation

For many, the most difficult aspect of dealing with an injury is not expending the psychic energy to recuperate, but rather, having to put up with a lower activity level while healing takes place. Long periods of inactivity can drive an athlete crazy while he or she chomps at the bit to get back on the tennis court or the running track.

A problem arises when injured athletes are so impatient to get active again that they return to sports activity after an injury heals without rehabilitating the injured region. If a healing process has been lengthy, the injured area will most probably lose strength and tone, as will perhaps the rest of the body. Therefore, even though one is sidelined with an injury, every attempt to exercise should be made in order to keep in condition. When the injury is healed, that region of the body should be strengthened so that reinjury will not occur. This point is probably the most overlooked and forgotten aspect of the treatment of sports injuries. If a muscle is not exercised, it rapidly loses strength—strength that must be replaced before athletic activity commences again. Chapter 6 describes exercises designed to recapture and improve muscle strength.

Not enough can be said for the strengthening of muscles and limbering of tendons to prevent athletic injury and reinjury. If muscles are strong and tendons flexible, they have a better chance to withstand the demands placed on them during sports activity. If people were in better shape, a lot of sports injuries would be avoided. We get into trouble when we ask our bodies to do things they once might have done but have not done for a long time.

Running through an Injury

There is conflicting opinion about the advisability of "running through" or "playing through" an injury. The conflict arises because sometimes it works and sometimes it does not. If you develop an ache or a pain and are not seriously hampered by it, you might try to continue your sports activities, perhaps at a slightly reduced level, and see if your body repair mechanisms can work faster than your injury-worsening activities. You might try using support bandages or strapping your injured part with tape and icing the injury before and after activity to reduce the pain and swelling. Be advised, however, that artifically supporting an injury can result in further and more serious damage because you will not be as aware of its resulting pain and discomfort.

25

Trying to "run through" or "play through" an injury is risky. If after a week or ten days the discomfort persists, stop your activity. Rest is usually the best remedy for a sports injury. Perhaps you'll want to consult a sports-injury specialist.

3 Types of Common Sports Injuries

Injury to some part of the primary movement system usually is the result of a severe stress placed on a muscle, tendon, ligament, or joint. The stress can be from a blow, such as getting kicked in the leg during a football game; or it can be the exertion of an abnormally strong pulling or twisting force on a muscle, tendon, or ligament that tears the fibers and perhaps ruptures some of the smaller associated blood vessels.

There are many types of sports injury; some are relatively benign, whereas others are serious enough to require hospitalization. Some injuries occur to one or more parts of the primary movement system and are therefore internal. Other injuries, such as cuts, scrapes, blisters, and rashes, are external. Injuries to specific body regions are discussed in chapters 7 to 11, and skin maladies are taken up in chapter 12.

This chapter deals with general types of sports injury regardless of the body region that is affected.

Contusions

There is hardly a person in the world who has not been bruised. And that is particularly true for athletes. Getting hit with a baseball, getting accidentally kicked in soccer, or falling down in a volleyball game all produce that characteristic sore place which frequently turns the skin black-and-blue.

In the jargon of sports medicine, traumatic blows to the body are *compression injuries,* and the damage they produce is called a *contusion,* which most people call a bruise.

A contusion involves the accumulation of tissue debris, blood, and other fluids that leak from damaged muscle and broken blood vessels. Normally, the blood clots to form a hematoma, and depending on the extent of the damage, will cause local pain, discolor the overlying skin, and impede function.

The treatment of a contusion varies depending on its severity, although in all cases the immediate treatment triad of ice, compression, and elevation is recommended. After the initial I.C.E. treatment, a mild contusion may require little more than a day or two of rest. However, moderate to severe contusions usually require additional treatment *after the internal bleeding stops*. Such treatment consists of warm-water soaks or whirlpool or jacuzzi treatments with a water temperature of about ninety degrees Fahrenheit, twice daily for fifteen minutes; an elastic wrap for support; and mild stretching.

It is imperative not to start the heat treatments too soon, or fluids may continue to leak into the injured region and healing time may be prolonged.

Even the worst contusions improve considerably in a couple of weeks, and then the athlete can return to activity.

Muscle-Tendon Strains or Pulls

Muscle-tendon strains or pulls happen frequently in sprint events at track meets. A typical situation can occur as follows: the runners explode out of the starting blocks and the runner who is third begins to make a move on the leaders when all of a sudden he or she pulls up lame and stops. A grimace of excruciating pain appears on the face, and a hand clutches the back of one of the thighs. More than likely the athlete has just suffered the agony of a pulled hamstring. Or, to be medically correct, a strained hamstring.

The runner has asked the knee flexors to do more than they are capable of, and the fibers of one (or more) of the hamstring group of muscles have torn. There was simply too much resistance to their pulling ability, and that runner is now out of commission for several weeks while the swelling and pain subside and the muscles knit.

The overstretching, tearing, or ripping of a muscle or its tendon is called a *strain*. The damage can range from tearing a few muscle or tendon fibers to complete rupturing of a muscle or even complete pulling away of a tendon from the bone to which it is attached, which is called an *avulsion*. Strains tend to occur in the weakest part of a muscle-tendon unit.

What causes strains? There is debate among sports-medicine experts about the answer, but it is obvious that it has something to do with muscle weakness. A muscle might be fatigued or might have lost necessary minerals through perspiration. The muscle-tendon unit might be much weaker than the muscle that opposes its action (the antagonist). One reason hamstring pulls occur so frequently is that the knee-extensor system (the quadriceps muscles in the thigh) is usually much stronger than the knee-flexor system (the hamstrings); this imbalance putting tremendous burdens on the flexors to keep pace with activity.

Immediate treatment for a strain is the same as that for a contusion: ice, compression, and elevation.

If there is near-complete or complete loss of function—for example, if bending at a joint is no longer possible—then medical advice should be sought immediately. Complete ruptures or avulsions sometimes require surgical treatment to restore the integrity of the muscle-tendon unit. Otherwise, after the initial stages of internal bleeding have stopped, one can facilitate the repair process with heat treatments and mild stretching within the limits of pain. Later, the entire musculo-tendon unit must be rehabilitated before activity resumes, or reinjury is all too likely.

Chronic Strain

Chronic Strain, caused by repeated low-grade strain of a muscle, tendon, or joint is a mild and continuous inflammation of that region characterized by local pain, point tenderness, swelling, and perhaps weakness.

When the inflammation involves tendons or muscle-tendon units,

29

it is called *tendinitis*. When the lubricating sheath surrounding a tendon is inflamed, the condition is referred to as *tenosynovitis*. Anyone afflicted with either of these conditions cares little about the distinction. When the lubricating sac, or *bursa,* that surrounds a joint becomes inflamed, large amounts of fluid are produced, filling the sac and causing pain and swelling. This condition is known as *bursitis*.

Treatment of these long-term chronic conditions involves rest, superficial heat treatments (such as using a heating pad or whirlpool a couple of times a day), and gradual stretching. Several weeks of treatment may be necessary to acquire normal, painless function again.

Rehabilitation should be undertaken to prevent the recurrence of the stress that initially caused the tendinitis or bursitis. This should be obvious. If the cause of the injurious condition is not corrected, it simply will recur. Sometimes surgery is necessary to repair the faulty anatomical conditions that bring on the condition.

Sprains

Sprains are partial or complete tears of ligaments that usually result in destablization of a joint. If the ligamentous support of a joint is damaged in such a way that the bones are no longer in their proper alignment, the joint is said to be dislocated. The ankles, knees, and shoulders are the most frequently sprained joints.

Immediate treatment of a sprain is, once again, I.C.E. Follow-up therapy involves heat treatments, support, and rest. The repair process may take six to eight weeks. Be sure to give it time, or the ligaments may not fully knit and the joint will be chronically weak. Strengthening the muscles around a joint can often provide protection against sprains and help stabilize a joint already weakened by a previous sprain.

Chronic ligament injury can often produce *arthritis,* a common legacy of many a professional football career.

Fractures

A *fracture* is a break in a bone. Sometimes the break is not

30

complete—the bone may only be cracked. In some cases the bone is completely parted—in one or more places.

If the broken ends of a fractured bone remain within the body, the fracture is said to be *simple*. If, however, the broken bone protrudes through the skin, the fracture is said to be *compound*.

If a bone is broken, or you suspect a bone is broken, do not attempt to administer I.C.E. or any other form of first aid unless the person is bleeding profusely or not breathing. In particular, do not move the broken arm or leg. Keep the injured body part still or you might make things worse. Get immediate medical attention.

The medical treatment of a fracture always entails first an X-ray examination to determine the nature and extent of the fracture. The next step is the realignment of the ends of the broken bones, called *setting* the bones. Once realigned, the fractured bones will be immobilized in a splint or cast until healing is complete—usually in about eight weeks.

Part 2

Preventing Sports Injuries

4 Be in Shape

Most people participate in amateur sports because (1) they want to have fun, (2) they want to do something well so that they can gain a sense of accomplishment, and (3) they want to feel physically and psychologically better. And while pursuing these goals, no one wants to be hurt.

It turns out that maximizing the fun/do well/feel good aspects of sports and minimizing the potential for injury go together. Participation in sports is most satisfying when you are concentrating on your sports activity so much that you are totally absorbed into it, when your body responds fluidly to your commands, when you run or play with impeccable form, and when your equipment and the playing field or court conditions are the best.

Sports injuries occur most often when you are tired, your muscles and joints are stiff, you are not into what you're doing, your equipment is faulty, or you play and move with poor form. Therefore, by taking your sports activity seriously enough to get the most enjoyment from it, you will also help minimize the likelihood of becoming injured.

Body Awareness

Because we live in a machine age, it is common to think of the

35

body as a special type of machine somehow separate from our sense of self—a machine that we have to control with our brain much as we control a car. In sports this notion leads to the idea that the best athletes are the people who consciously control their body the most effectively. But if you ask good athletes what they experience when they are "doing their sports thing," they will not tell you that when they are performing they have to think very hard about making every movement accurate and precise. Instead, they will tell you that when they are at their best they are not thinking at all about what their bodies are doing. They simply "let it happen." Their minds and bodies seem to merge into an organic whole. The idea of the mind operating a separate control over the body machine does not apply.

The point is that sports performance requires recognition of the body not as a separate machine but as an integral part of yourself. Not enough can be said about the positive effect of this *holistic* attitude in avoiding sports injuries (and staying healthy otherwise, too). An integrated approach to the workings of the mind and body is the first requisite to enjoyable and injury-free sports activity.

Learn to listen to your body. Get to know it as you would a very special, personal friend. One way to do that is to take a ten-minute period of time each day to practice a body-awareness exercise. Do the exercise in a quiet place and wear clothes in which you feel comfortable. Begin by lying down on your back (on a soft surface or a blanket) with your arms at your sides, palms facing up, and your feet slightly apart (about twelve inches). Close your eyes, breathe normally, and then begin a private conversation with your body.

Focus attention on your feet and lower legs and notice if there's any stiffness or pain, or, on the other hand, if they feel great. Do that with all the parts of your body, one region at a time, until you have surveyed your entire body and you know how you are doing. Start with your feet and lower legs and then move to your upper legs. Then move on to the pelvic area, abdomen, chest, back, left shoulder, and arm; then the right shoulder and right arm, the neck, and finally, the face and head.

If there is a particularly tight place, focus on that region and concentrate on loosening it. Talk to it gently. Say, "Loosen up legs, that's right, now you're doing it. Get loose." Be sure not to come on like a tyrant or you will stiffen in addition to losing the connectedness this exercise is supposed to foster. Be gentle with yourself.

To loosen a particularly tight place, some people imagine that place to be a cube of sugar or a pat of butter. As they give themselves mental or verbal suggestions to relax that spot, they simultaneously imagine the sugarcube or butter melting, thus helping the tight spot to "disintegrate" into looseness.

Breathing is very important, too. While you are on your back, take a few deep breaths. Inhale slowly for a count of eight, filling your lungs completely. Hold the air inside for a two-count and then exhale over another eight-count. As you inhale think to yourself that you are taking in good air and upon exhaling that you are getting rid of bad air. Imagine the good air, containing life-giving oxygen, going to the various parts of your body, which when reaching a particularly tight or sore place, brings fortifying and healing energy that is capable of positively affecting that place.

After merely a few of these sessions you will begin to notice what your body is "saying to you"—whether you are stiff, sore, tired, neutral, loose, or raring-to-go. Learn to listen to your body. You will like what you hear.

Learning to listen to your body has all-important consequences when you are participating in sports. You will be able to tell when you can exert to the fullest of, and even beyond, your previous limit, which is tremendously exhilarating. And you will be able to know when you're too tired to push. How many skiers' injuries occur on the last run of the day when the legs are too tired to control the skis? Runners must be particularly aware, for they have to learn to distinguish between their psychological reluctance to run on certain days, which manifests itself as fatigue, and actual muscle tiredness. A long or strenuous run on tired legs might result in severe leg cramps, or worse, a strained tendon.

Exertion is good, but overwork is foolhardy. Learn to listen to your body and use your common sense.

Being in Shape

Whatever your sport, it will be to your benefit if your overall level of fitness is as high as you can attain. By being in good shape you'll feel better, have more endurance in both sports and nonsports activity; improve your health by improving heart, lung, and circulatory function; and increase the likelihood of remaining injury-free. Your muscles will be stronger and tendons and ligaments flexible enough to be able to take the stresses of sports activity, and your increased endurance will keep you from getting hurt due to fatigue.

Although you may play squash three times a week or jog every morning, unless you get your heart rate above 130 to 140 beats per minute for a few minutes each day you are not likely to be getting any training effect from your efforts. That does not mean that your exercise level is a waste, but it does mean that you should not have any illusions about being in good shape either. If your level of activity makes you sweat and your heart pound, however, then you are probably giving yourself a reasonably good workout.

If you decide to embark on a training program, you should plan what you are going to do very carefully. Impulsively running three miles one day to work yourself into shape in a hurry is not likely to ensure increased physical fitness. More often than not, it is likely to wipe you out so much that you will never want to run again. Whether you choose a training program that involves running, swimming, cycling, or lifting, there are some guidelines you would do well to follow.

Physical checkup. With the epidemic interest in amateur sports and physical fitness, most doctors are becoming knowledgeable about the risks of suddenly increasing the level of physical activity. If you are contemplating a dramatic increase in your activity level, consult a sports-minded physician who can give your heart, lungs, and body a good checkup to make sure you aren't likely to harm yourself.

Enjoy what you're doing. Too often, people have the expectation that exercise must be psychologically and physically painful if it is to be beneficial. For some, the idea of training is as attractive as going to war. It is true that you should breathe and exert yourself beyond previous limits, but at the same time you don't have to kill yourself. Sports are supposed to be fun; they are supposed to make you feel good.

So make your training enjoyable. Choose activities you like. That way you are likely to continue with your program. If you feel being around people will make your activity more fun, join a class or organize some friends so that you can work out together. After you have had a particularly good workout, or whenever you exceed a previous limit, reward yourself. Pat yourself on the back and compliment yourself on doing well. Remind yourself that you are a good person and that you have done a hard thing and are deserving of recognition.

Do not fall into the trap of thinking that sports activity must involve competition. The emphasis placed on competition in sports in our culture too often overlooks the personally gratifying qualities of physical activity: to improve one's sense of health and well-being and to have fun. Give yourself permission to participate in sports without the need to be competitive, unless, of course, you want to be.

Accomplish goals. The guiding principle of any training program is to work toward improving one's performance. So set some goals for yourself—only be sure they are ones that you can attain. If you have done nothing athletic for a long time, then set a goal of jogging or swimming for a minute without stopping. Then progress to two minutes when you think your body is ready to undertake the challenge. That may be in a day or it may be a week. Take your time. Getting into shape cannot happen overnight.

People in training need a plan—a well-conceived program that will help them achieve their fitness goals. Devising such plans is the province of coaches, although anyone can make up a plan that is personally suitable. If you want a fitness plan, you can consult the local high school coach, read any number of "how-to" books for particular sports, or follow the plan outlined in Dr. Kenneth Cooper's book, *The New Aerobics*.

It is customary in our culture to measure performance by "how fast" and "how far." That's well and good for some things, such as the progress of people involved in heavy competition. Speed and distance are not necessarily the best goals for amateurs who put sports into their lives in order to receive greater enjoyment from living. For these people, more personal goals such as "does this level of activity make me feel good?" or "does this help me with my goal of losing weight?" make more sense than blind adherence to a stopwatch.

Progress slowly. The best way to get into shape is to do it with moderation. If you push too hard too fast, you are likely to get fatigued to the point that you will not want to continue. Even worse, you may injure yourself, perhaps seriously.

Use your common sense and progress in moderation.

Warm up and cool down. How many people warm up their car engines before they drive on the highway but do not warm up their bodies before playing two or three sets of tennis? After waiting for a court and knowing that other players are waiting for you to finish, it's too tempting to peel off one's sweats and dash onto the court to begin hard play. This is foolhardy.

All sports activity should be preceded by at least a five-minute period of warm-up that includes stretching, breathing, relaxation, and easy running. It is imperative that the muscles and tendons become loose before activity begins, or injury might result. Ideally, one should undertake an exercise program that affects all regions of the body. Some exercises that are particularly good are suggested in Chapter 6.

When you are finished with your training or sports activity, it is a good idea to let the body cool down slowly. You should walk or jog easily while the heart and lungs return to their normal physiological activity level. You should breathe normally to repay the oxygen debt built up by exercise. And you should stretch muscles and tendons before hitting the showers.

Exercise regularly. It is better not to exercise at all than it is to exercise hard intermittently. Without the progressive buildup of

40

strength and cardiorespiratory efficiency that comes from regular physical activity, the strains on body tissues are too great and injury may result.

5 Improving Flexibility and Form

One of the best ways to avoid sports injuries is to improve your body's flexibility—your ability to bend, straighten, and twist. Studies have shown that athletes who commit themselves to improving flexibility have fewer injuries. Flexibility also contributes to feeling healthy, which is true even for nonathletes.

Achieving flexibility requires a persistent, almost daily routine of stretching the muscles, tendons, and ligaments of the body. If the stretching isn't practiced regularly, the gains made will be nullified by periods of inactivity.

In elementary school or high school many people learned the *ballistic* (bouncing) method of stretching. Touching the toes (an exercise to stretch the hamstring group of muscles in the back of the thigh) involved bending forward with the arms outstretched and bouncing at the waist, trying to touch the ground. With each "bounce" one was supposed to reach closer to the ground.

At the present time the ballistic method is no longer recommended by many trainers, coaches, and athletes. It has been replaced by the *static* method, which entails gradually stretching to, and then past, the point of discomfort, holding the longest possible stretch for thirty seconds to a minute. The ballistic method has lost favor because it produces a reflex tightening of the muscles and apparently causes some slight muscle damage.

When you want to stretch your hamstrings, you should sit on the floor with the legs extended and bend at the waist, trying to touch the toes. You should keep bending and stretching as far as possible until the "point of discomfort." That is recognizable by feeling low-level pain as the muscles reluctantly give up their tightness. Do not stop the stretch at the point of discomfort, but hold it for a few seconds; the discomfort will subside and you will be able to stretch further. Keep stretching until you either reach your goal of stretching for so many seconds or until the point of sharp or intense pain. At that point you can relax and take a deep breath or two.

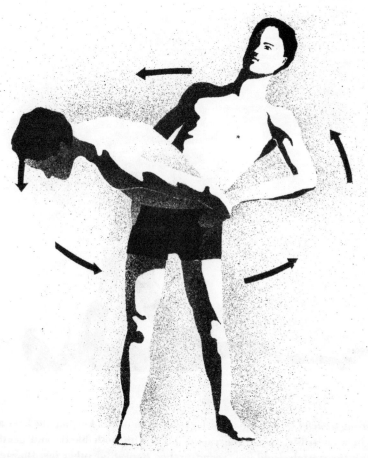

Trunk circling. **Take five seconds to circle clockwise; relax. Repeat in counterclockwise direction. Do each direction at least twice.**

Many athletes have adopted the postures of Hatha Yoga to use as flexibility increasers and muscle toners. If you are interested in applying these useful and centuries-old techniques, you can buy any of a number of yoga instruction books, join a yoga class at your local YMCA, church, or school, or you can watch Lilias Folan, the yoga instructor on public television. Lilias also has a yoga instruction book that is available through most public television stations.

If you are athletically active on a regular basis and have not done so already, it is a good idea to incorporate a regime of flexibility exercises into your activity. Several fundamental stretching exer-

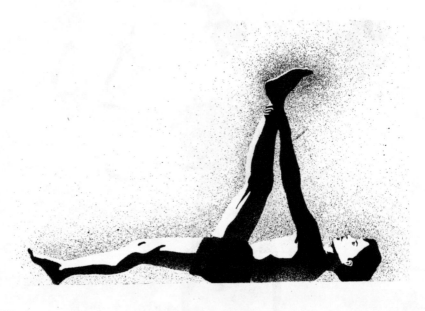

Hamstring stretch I. Slowly raise one leg to an angle of 90°, keeping the knee as straight as possible. Grasp the raised ankle with both hands and gently increase the stretch. Hold five seconds; relax. Repeat for other leg. Do each leg twice.

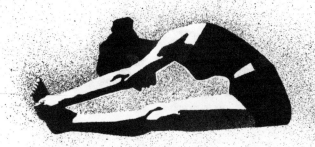

Hamstring stretch II. Bend at the waist holding onto toes or ankles. Attempt to place head on knees, hold thirty or sixty seconds.

cises are illustrated in the accompanying diagrams. Most people do their stretching exercises immediately before they work out or play, but others who are on stricter schedules manage to do their stretching in a fifteen-minute span at some other time of the day.

A comprehensive exercise routine would include almost all of those illustrated, and perhaps it would include muscle-strengthening exercises for specific body regions as well (see chapter 6). Here are two sample flexibility programs:

Flexibility Program for Running:
1. Walk or run easily for one quarter of a mile
2. Hamstring stretch I
3. Abdominal stretch I
4. Abductor stretch
5. Groin stretch
6. Hamstring stretch II
7. Push-up
8. Hurdle stretch
9. Gastrocnemius stretch

Flexibility Program for Tennis and other racketsports:
1. Trunk circling
2. Hamstring stretch II
3. Groin stretch
4. Abdominal stretch II

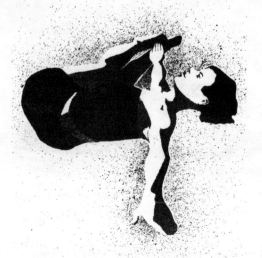

Abdominal stretch I. **Lie on back with arms in "T" position. Raise both legs to 90°. Lower legs to touch right hand, hold five seconds. Raise legs to starting position, hold five seconds. Lower legs to touch left hand, hold five seconds. Raise legs, hold five seconds. Lower legs and relax. Repeat entire exercise.**

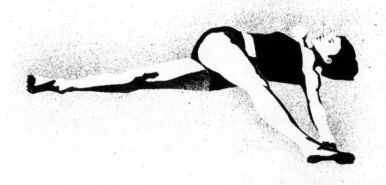

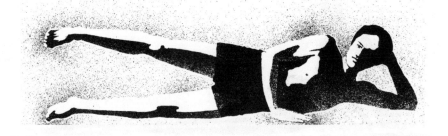

Abductor stretch. **Lift leg to the point of resistance, hold thirty second; relax.**

5. Push-up
6. Ski stretch
7. Gastrocnemius stretch
8. Run in place for one minute
9. Jump in place for one minute
10. Practice strokes—ten each of forehands, backhands, and overheads

If you choose to design a flexibility program for yourself, be sure to include at least one abdominal-, one hamstring-, and one gastrocnemius-stretching exercise.

And if you are already in the habit of stretching before you work out, be aware that it is also advisable to do a few stretching exercises after your activity to prevent stiffness. Often a good hamstring stretch is enough.

Abdominal stretch II. **Lie on back with arms in "T" position. Raise left leg to 90° keeping knee straight. Lower left leg across the body to touch right hand; hold five seconds. Raise leg to 90° position, then relax. Repeat for right leg, crossing over to touch the left hand. Do exercise twice.**

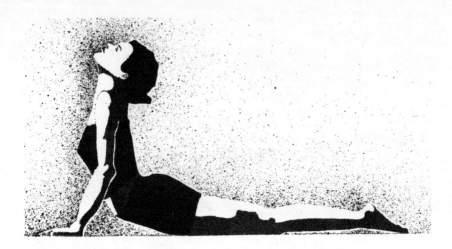

Cobra posture. Lie face down with hands under shoulders. With forehead on floor, slowly raise forehead, then nose, then chin, then shoulders, upper and middle back. Take ten seconds to complete extension; hold extension five seconds. Relax.

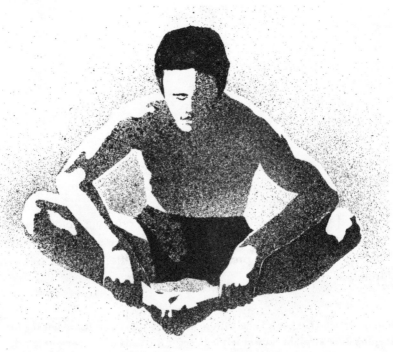

Groin stretch. Assume stretch position and pull ankles toward the body to increase the stretch on groin muscles.

48

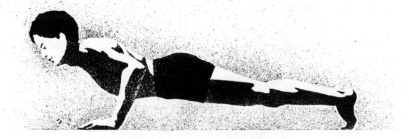

Push-up. Do at least thirty.

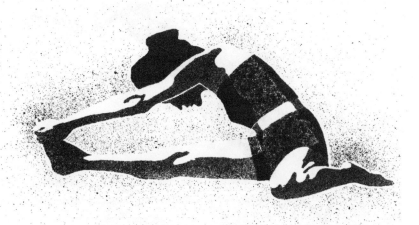

Hurdle stretch. Keep knee straight. Hold thirty seconds.

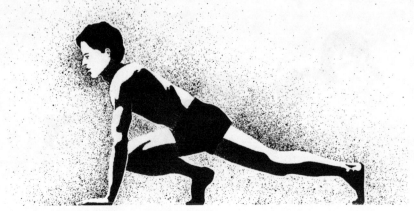

Ski stretch. **Hold thirty seconds.**

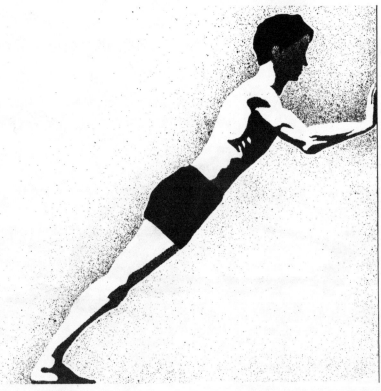

Gastrocnemius stretch. **Lean against a wall at an angle of between 45° and 60°. Keeping heels on the floor, lean closer to the wall. Hold fifteen seconds. Relax.**

Form

No sport is fun if your form is bad. If you do not do it right, whether it is swinging a racket, throwing a ball, or running, you will not do it well and won't enjoy what you are doing as much as those whose form is good. Moreover, you may be vulnerable to injury.

Proper form is best learned from a qualified instructor. If you think your style needs improvement, get yourself a private teacher, take a class at the local YMCA, community center, or playground, or read a "how to" book. Schools and colleges offer an array of fitness and sports classes. Just telephone the athletic department and ask for information about sports programs for the public.

Beware of advice from your fellow jocks. Misinformation, superstition, and private theories permeate "jockdom." Before you heed any suggestions, be sure that the advice you receive has withstood the test of producing successful athletes.

6 Strengthen Muscles

Sports medicine experts agree that the most important factor in avoiding sports injuries is muscle strength. Strong muscles are able to perform commands given to them without the stress of overwork, and they can continue to work without fatigue for the time period that one is active.

College and professional athletes spend many hours conditioning their bodies in order to improve their athletic performance and also stay injury-free. They go through carefully designed training regimens that may include a muscle-strengthening program of weight lifting, special muscle-building exercises, exercises to improve endurance, and activities that improve flexibility.

Most amateur jocks cannot devote the same time and energy to a rigorous training program as do college and professional athletes. It is just too hard to budget the psychological space among all the other demands for time and attention made by job, family, and just plain living. Tennis is tennis, however, requiring the same start-and-stop running and ball-hitting motions whether you are Jimmy Connors or unseeded in your local tennis tournament. And if you are not as strong as a pro, your risk for injury is greater.

Although it may seem unreasonable, every amateur should realize that ideally, he or she ought to build the muscle strength and endurance of a pro in order to avoid injury. If that cannot be done, one should do one's best to approximate that level, given present life circumstances and athletic goals.

Rehabilitation

For amateur athletes, perhaps the most overlooked aspect of injury prevention is increasing the muscle strength of an injured region after healing has taken place. The problem is that when the repair process is complete, people mistakenly think the injured region is "normal" again and they can resume their full preinjury sports regimen. In one sense this is true, for torn muscle, tendon, or ligament fibers have mended, blood vessels have repaired, pain and swelling are gone, and the injured part can move again. But often what is not realized is that while the healing process was taking place, the injured region (and perhaps the rest of the body) was inactive and hence losing strength, flexibility, and tone. Therefore, even when the repair process is complete, the injured region is weak from inactivity, although it may be structurally intact. And, since muscle strength is the most effective prevention of sports injury, the weakened post-injured body is much more vulnerable to injury than before.

Therefore, before returning to activity it is imperative that the injured region be rehabilitated to restore former strength and if possible, exceed it, since presumably it was weakness in that region that permitted the injury to occur in the first place.

Muscle Strengthening Exercises

The usual way to increase muscle strength is to perform specific exercises designed to improve a particular region of the body. Some standard exercises are pictured at the end of this chapter.

Most people do not have the time to follow a thorough exercise program, so they have to select the few exercises that are likely to do them the most good. Here are some suggestions for abbreviated exercise plans:

RUNNING

Most runners suffer from lower leg and knee problems, so exercises designed to strengthen the leg muscles are most important. The heel raise builds strength in the calf and helps protect the Achilles tendon and other leg tendons, and the knee extension and stair run help develop the quadriceps, which protects the knees.

TENNIS

Probably half of America's amateur tennis players have elbow and arm problems; therefore, they should devote energy to building forearm strength by squeezing a tennis ball a few minutes each day. Another important exercise for tennis players is plantar flexion. It will help strengthen the ankles.

SKIING

Downhill skiing puts great demands on the knees and hips. The stair run is an excellent exercise for skiers, for not only does it build strength in the upper legs, which helps protect the knees from damage, but it also increases aerobic capacity and thereby increases endurance. Another good knee exercise is the knee extender, which should be done while wearing ski boots. Hip circling will help prevent strains to the hip joint.

There are some points to consider when doing these exercises:

1. Ideally, each exercise should be performed two or three times a day, particularly if the goal of the exercise is to rehabilitate a once-injured region.
2. Each exercise should be repeated until the ultimate goal of three sets of ten repetitions each set is reached.
3. Do all the exercises smoothly (no bouncing or jerking).
4. Do the exercises within the limits of pain, remembering that overcoming resistance and discomfort are part of muscle building.

One additional point to remember: professional and college athletes have the encouragement of coaches, trainers, and teammates to help them pursue their exercise programs diligently. The amateur, often without such a vast support system, must rely on self-discipline and inner motivation to accomplish athletic goals. One simply has to keep with it no matter how lonely or boring it may seem.

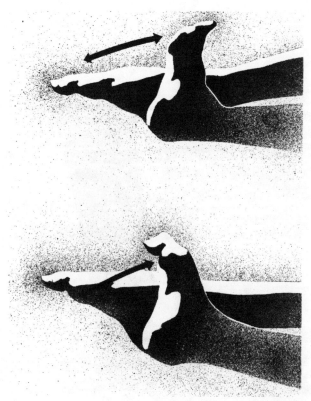

Plantar Flexion and Dorsiflexion. **Bend foot up, hold five seconds, relax; bend foot down, hold five seconds, relax.**

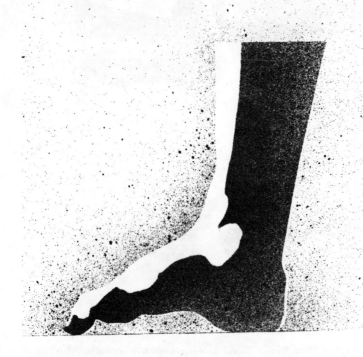

Foot arch. **Hold five seconds; relax.**

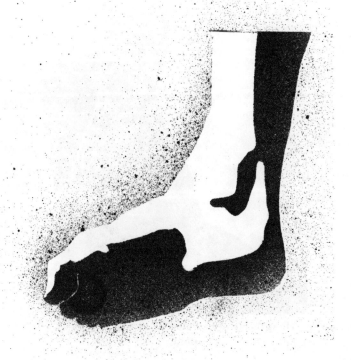

Marble pick up. **Hold five seconds, relax. Work up to ten repetitions.**

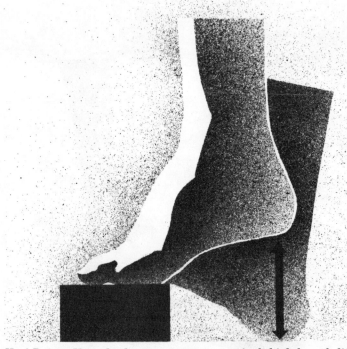

Heel Raises. Hang heels over a step or two-inch-high board, lift onto toes; relax. Work up to thirty repetitions.

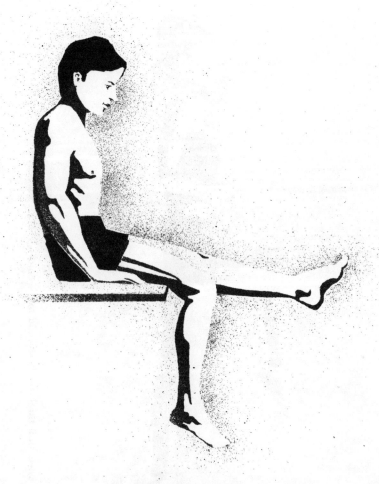

Knee Extension. Straighten leg, hold ten seconds; relax. Work up to thirty repetitions shoeless, then with shoes, and finally with five-pound weights.

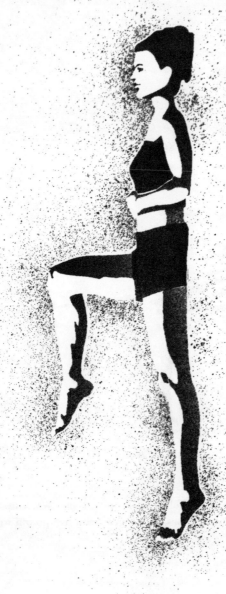

Quadriceps Stretch. **Bend knee, pull thigh to chest, hold five seconds, relax.**

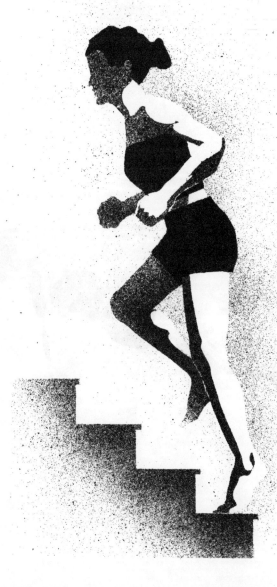

Stair run. **Run up twenty (or more) stairs, jog or walk down. Repeat five times. Work up to ten minutes duration.**

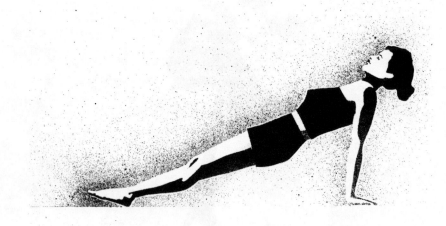

Hip Lift. **Hold five seconds, relax.**

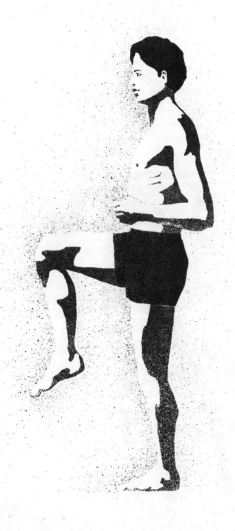

Hip Flexion. Raise thigh to abdomen, hold five seconds, relax. Work up to five-pound weight or boot.

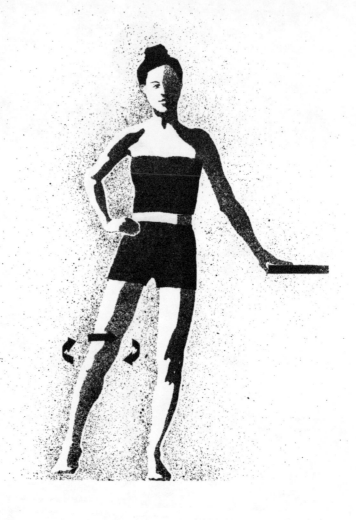

Hip Circling. **Rotate leg ten seconds.**

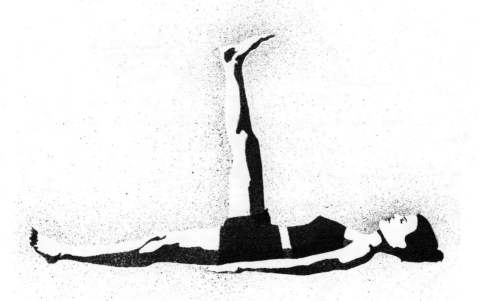

Leg Lift. **Lift leg. Hold five seconds, relax.**

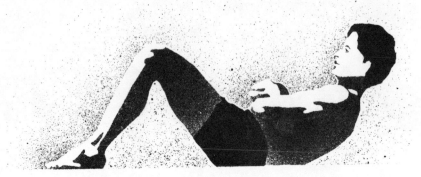

Abdominal Curl. **Fold arms across chest; lift shoulders and hold five seconds; relax.**

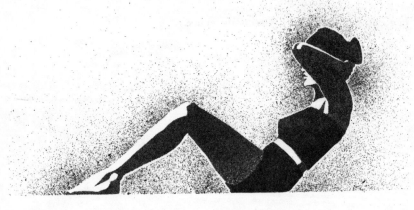

Sit-Up. **Work up to thirty.**

66

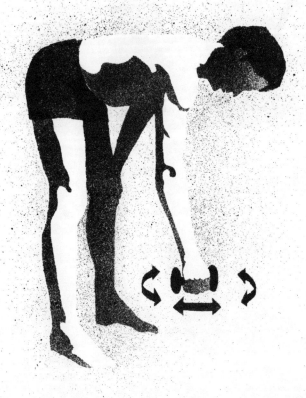

Pendulum. Swing arm across the body in a pendulum motion holding a five-pound weight. Work up to fifty repetitions.

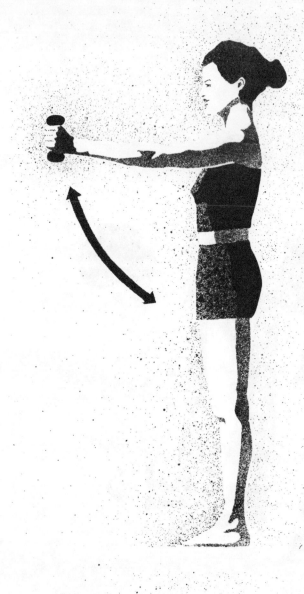

Arm Raise. **Raise arm, hold parallel to floor five seconds, relax. Work up to thirty repetitions with five-pound weight.**

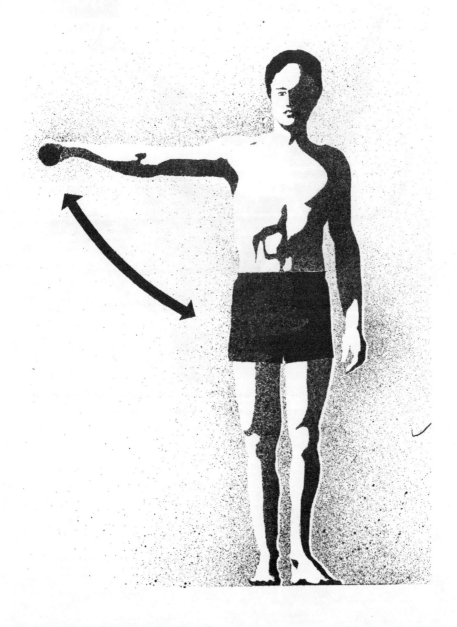

Abduction Raise. Raise arm, hold at side five seconds, relax. Work up to thirty repetitions with five-pound weight.

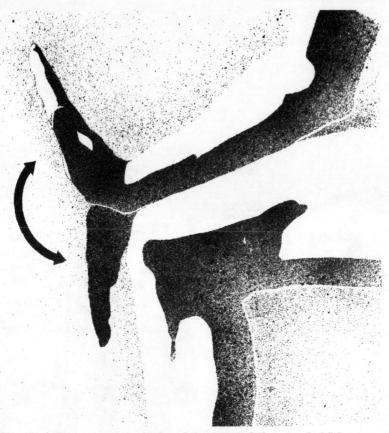

Wrist Curl. Place arms on thighs while sitting. Lift wrist, hold five seconds, relax. Work up to thirty repetitions with five-pound weight.

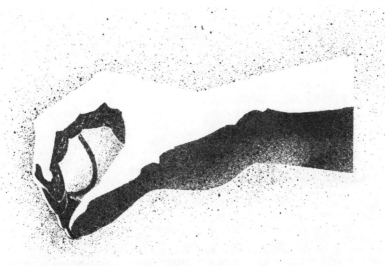

Ball Squeeze. Squeeze a tennis ball or rubber ball very hard fifty times.

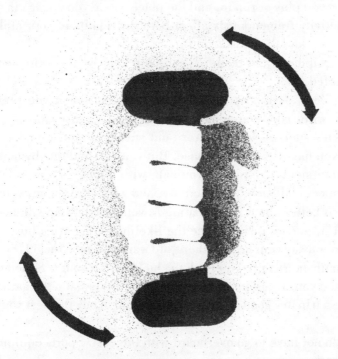

Wrist Twist. Twist wrist slowly back and forth for ten seconds, relax. Work up to five repetitions with five-pound weight.

7 Use Good Equipment

There is no doubt that the equipment you use, the clothes you wear, the shoes you play or run in, and the place where you engage in your sports activity tremendously affect both the quality of your athletic performance and the satisfaction you receive from sports. Moreover, proper equipment and facilities can help keep you healthy and off the disabled list.

Regardless of your sport, you will enjoy it more if you provide yourself with good equipment. It is easy to use inexpensive equipment, such as your old worn-out sneakers, and whatever old clothes you have around the house. But you will find that by making the commitment to provide yourself with proper shoes, clothes chosen specifically for sports activity, and good equipment, you will feel much better about participating in your sport. You will also do better at it, and you will reduce the likelihood of getting hurt.

So throw away your grandfather's old warped tennis racket (or save it as a family heirloom), give back the hickory skis your 6'8" neighbor has loaned you, toss your old high school sneakers into the garbage, and take a trip to a good sports outfitting shop to buy the best you can afford.

You do not have to go overboard with the cost. Sports equipment can be rather expensive, so use your common sense. Be a smart shopper.

Before you plunk any money down, make the sales people in the shop tell you the good and bad points about the different brands of equipment you are interested in. Perhaps shop at several stores just to get an idea of who knows best. Ask your friends what experiences they have had with their equipment. For that matter, ask any jock-type who you think might have a worthwhile opinion. All jocks like to be asked their "professional" opinion. And it is a certainty that every jock—professional or amateur, has one. By all means, don't be afraid to ask.

When buying equipment there are some points to consider:
1. How will the equipment be used? In what climate? How often? On what kind of surface? For fun only or in competition, or both? Be sure to discuss these factors with your consultants before you buy.
2. How many seasons will you get from your new gear? Once you acquire something that you like it is certain that you will want to keep it. Therefore, be sure it will last and also find out if it can be repaired.
3. Be wary of new products or models unless you can assure yourself that they do what they are supposed to.

Shoes

Good athletic shoes are probably the most important investment you can make. There are several well-known sports-shoe manufacturers, such as Adidas, Nike, Puma, Spot-Bilt, Converse, Tiger, and Tretorn, as well as other good ones that are not so well-known. Each company may have several styles and designs, therefore, it is best to have a knowledgeable salesperson at a sports-shoe store help you choose the best shoe for your particular feet and athletic needs.

If you are buying shoes for tennis or other court sports, try to buy them from someone who plays tennis. The same holds true for running. Rely on a salesperson only if personal experience is one of the bases of his or her advice. Do not buy shoes from a regular shoe dealer unless you have confidence in that person's knowledge about the needs of athletes. And never buy sports shoes in the supermarket because they are inexpensive. Be prepared to spend about $30 for a good pair of sports shoes, which is cheap considering how important they are.

When buying athletic shoes, the foremost considerations are support and proper fit. Remember, the feet bear the entire body weight and they have to withstand a lot of pounding and twisting in athletic activity. They want to do their job, but if you do not give them a break they will rebel by hurting, transmitting shocks and jars to the knee and hip and thereby make them sore, and cause blisters, corns, bunions, hammer toes, and painful or fallen arches to develop.

Utilizing the principle of outfitting yourself properly and with good sense, be sure to use shoes that are designed specifically for your sport. Sports-shoe companies hire professional athletes, coaches, and knowledgeable sports medicine experts to help them design the best shoes possible that take into account features such as support, durability, and traction. Anyone who has gotten sore, tired feet from trying to play tennis in running shoes knows that "a sports shoe is not a *sports* shoe." The same is true of people who have repeatedly tried to run long distances in tennis shoes. Running shoes have a relatively narrow sole designed especially for the straightforward foot-plants of a runner, whereas tennis and other court-sport shoes have a wider sole to take into account that the demands of a player are stops and starts, sudden changes of direction, and jumping. Moreover, running shoes do not offer the lateral support that court-sport shoes do.

Features to look for in both running and court-sport shoes are a well-constructed arch for foot comfort and ligament support and a cushion sole to absorb shocks from the running or playing surface. Shoes with two-layered soles—one of a soft, spongy material for shock absorption and the other of a harder rubbery material for stability—are best. The upper part of the shoe can be made of soft nylon, leather, or canvas—whichever is your preference. Shoes with nylon uppers hold their shape after getting wet better than shoes of canvas or leather, but they are not as porous and therefore they do not allow the feet to "breathe." Some people prefer to use shoes with high tops, for they give additional ankle support.

Once you have selected the make and model of the shoes just right for your needs, you have to be sure that they fit properly. Most people's feet are not of equal size, and because sports shoes do not come in the wide varieties of sizes that street shoes do, achieving the proper fit requires some attention and care.

When fitting shoes, wear the socks you will actually be wearing with those shoes. Then try on the shoes and notice if there are any pinching sensations around the toes or on the sides of the feet. There should be enough room for your toes to move and even spread a little, and your longest toe (either the big toe or the second toe) should have about one-half inch of space from the front of the shoe. The widest part of the shoe should fit precisely the widest part of your foot. The shoe should be flexible and bend or "break" at the widest part of your foot, not in front and not behind.

Put both shoes of a pair on, lace them up as you would for actual use, and then try them out right there in the shop. Run around in them, jump a few times, change directions quickly to see if your foot slips at all. Then try on a pair the next size larger, or perhaps a pair from a different manufacturer. Considering how important these shoes are, it is to your advantage to be sure that they are exactly right for you.

Fitting spiked or cleated shoes requires the application of these same principles. One additional consideration is that studies have indicated that the longer the cleat the higher the incidence of injury. Thus, shoes with short polyurethane cleats or those with a ridged sole are probably better than shoes with long metal cleats or spikes.

One of the hardest things you may ever have to do is discard your favorite shoes, particularly after they have helped you run hundreds of miles or win hundreds of matches. But when your sports shoes wear down, retire them. Enshrine them, or throw them out, but do not use them. If you continue to run or play with worn soles, you will put stresses and strains on the tendons of your leg muscles that may produce disabling and painful tendinitis. Or if the arch of the shoe starts to break down, the arch of your foot may be next.

Some jocks get so emotionally attached to their favorite shoes that they cannot bear to part with them. These intransigents can try to keep their shoes alive by having a sports-shoe repair expert (like the Tred-2 people) give the shoes a sole or arch transplant. Or, they can try to do the needed repair themselves. It is possible to buy gooey substances (called *Goo* or *Sole Saver*) that are plastered on a shoe to rebuild the sole. New arches can be constructed from Dr. Scholl's shoe inserts, surgical padding or moleskin, or foam rubber held in place with glue or tape.

Rebuilding the sole and/or arch may be a good idea with brand new shoes, too. It is a way to get custom-fitted sports shoes. People with fallen arches (flat feet) or people who have one leg longer than the other, (which can cause knee and hip problems in active athletes) may find custom remodeling of their shoes a necessity. To help design custom-rebuilt sports shoes, it is a good idea to consult a sports-minded podiatrist or shoemaker. Such custom-designed shoe alterations are called *orthotics*.

Socks

Wearing socks is a good idea regardless of your sport. They help prevent blisters.

Some trainers and coaches recommend wearing two pairs of socks, a pair of thin cotton socks underneath, and a thicker pair of wool or cotton-blend socks on top. Athletic socks should be white, because dyes (which may be harmful) tend to leach from colored socks and stain the feet.

It is important that socks fit properly, for friction from folds and wrinkles can cause blisters. Some people prefer to wear tubesocks because they have no sewn-in heel and therefore have no seam to cause irritation. On the other hand, some people prefer regular socks of the proper size, claiming that they fit more snugly than tubesocks and therefore offer even better protection against blisters.

Wool or thick cotton knee socks are beneficial for absorbing blows to the legs in basketball or soccer competition, and they also help retain body heat in the lower legs, which may reduce the risk of cramping and muscle strain.

Clothes

Your choice of sports clothes is totally up to you. Some people spend a great deal of money on the flashiest tennis clothes or nylon warm-up suits, and others "do their thing" in cut-offs and gray cotton

76

sweats. The important factor is not looks but comfort. If you feel good in your sports clothes you will probably improve your performance and most certainly will enjoy your sport more.

One possible problem that can be avoided by a wise choice in sports clothes is skin irritation. Cotton and wool absorb sweat better than nylon and, therefore, are less irritating when wet. That is why many athletes prefer cotton or cotton-blend clothes next to their skin from underwear out, thus presenting the irony of jocks not even wearing jocks. Perhaps the only time cotton clothes can be a problem is when they are worn in the rain; they get water-logged and seem to weigh a ton. Wool doesn't absorb water as much as cotton; therefore it is better to wear wool when it rains. Wearing a nylon shell over everything is a good idea, too.

If you work out or compete in very cold climates, be sure you insulate your body well with layers of clothes. Wear flannel thermal pants or pajama bottoms under your usual running pants and a sweatshirt or sweater over your usual running top. Be certain your hands and face are covered to prevent frostbite. By all means be sure to wear a hat or cap. The body gives up an enormous amount of heat through the scalp.

Facilities

Where you play or run is a crucial factor in preventing injuries. Basically, you will do fine if you use your common sense. If you're a runner, surfaces especially prepared for running—like college or high school tracks—are best. The key is to have a resilient, flat surface. Hard surfaces such as sidewalks and streets put tremendous strains on your feet and legs and should be avoided if possible. If you do run on cement, however, be sure to wear extra supportive shoes with super-shock-absorbing soles. Running on flat surfaces is essential because you reduce the risk of stepping into ruts and holes that may cause an ankel sprain or twisted knee. Also be aware that artificial grass surfaces like those in many professional sports stadiums contribute to more injuries than natural grass. The plastic of which they are made is hard and abrasive, so it is more conducive to contusions, sprains, and skin irritations than natural grass.

Artificial surfaces do have the advantage, however, of being free of gopher and sprinkler holes.

Braces and Tape

What about braces and tape? There is controversy about the advisability of using artificial support devices, especially for amateurs. Professional football players need all the help they can get, so they are often liberally taped and bandaged before they play. Serious weight lifters often wear special support belts. Other professional athletes use tape and bandages for support, often to reinforce a vulnerable place already weakened by injury.

The disadvantage of bandages and tape is that they tend to give a false sense of security. Someone might be fooled into thinking that by wearing a brace or by taping a limb, he or she is protected from getting hurt. That is not true. Since professional athletes are presumably already in peak condition, bandages and tape offer them a possible ounce of prevention in addition to a psychological boost in confidence. For an amateur who is not in very good shape, they offer little in the way of help. Remember, the best way to prevent athletic injuries is to increase muscle strength and joint flexibility. An elbow brace does not furnish the same protection against tennis elbow that strong forearm muscles do. And neither can a brace make up for a poor forehand ground stroke.

Unless a coach, trainer, or physician outfits you with some sort of brace, bandage, or tape, it is best not to depend on artificial supports to prevent sports injuries. It is better to concentrate on increasing your body strength and flexibility, and improving your form.

Part 3
Specific Sports Injuries

8 Foot and Ankle Problems

Foot and ankle problems are legion in sports activity. That is because the feet and ankles support the entire weight of the body, and they have to bear the brunt of all the twisting, pounding, and contorting that accompany athletic competition.

Foot Problems

The foot is made up of twenty-six bones. Fourteen of these are the bones of the toes. Another five comprise the middle of the foot; these are the *metatarsals*. The other seven bones make up the top and back of the foot. They are called the *tarsals*. Two of the tarsal bones are frequently involved in sports injuries. They are the *talus,* or ankle bone, and the *calcaneus,* or heel bone.

It has been estimated that in three sets of tennis a person takes up to 10,000 steps. And running for an hour involves about 5000. That is a lot of wear and tear on the feet, and so it is no wonder that many athletes are hampered by foot problems. Foot problems involving the skin—like blisters and athlete's foot—are discussed in chapter 12. The foot problems discussed here are structural problems caused by either improperly fitted shoes, continued stress from pounding the playing or running surface, and faulty posture.

Exostoses are abnormal outgrowths of one or more of the foot bones, most often caused by inflammation from poorly fitting shoes. Continual rubbing upon some part of the foot irritates the bone in that region to the degree that new bone is produced. Common sites of exostoses are on the outside of the foot just below the little toe and on the heel.

Some exostoses are relatively benign and give little trouble; others can become very painful and must be treated surgically. Assuming you have no hereditary predisposition for exostoses or any postural problems that bring them on, you can avoid them simply by being sure your shoes fit properly.

Bunions are abnormal outgrowths on the side of the foot just below the big toe and/or the little toe (called a tailor's bunion) that are usually very tender and painful. They are caused by ill-fitting shoes that produce chronic inflammation of the underlying bone and the bursal sac that covers it. The inflammation causes swelling, which in turn causes the tenderness and pain. By recognizing a bunion early in its development and having it taken care of, and by making sure your shoes fit well, you can probably avoid future bunions.

Hammer toes are the result of deformations in the toes caused by shoes that are too short. When such ill-fitting shoes are worn over a long period of time, they cramp the toes and cause them to assume a permanently bent position. Often corrective surgery is the only treatment. Prevention of hammer toes, of course, is assured by wearing shoes that fit properly.

An *ingrown toenail* usually occurs on the big toe. One reason for this is that the toenail tends to grow in a spiral fashion, and therefore it has a natural tendency to curve inward.

One can avoid ingrown toenails by being sure that shoes and socks fit properly and that toenails are correctly trimmed. When trimming the toenails be sure that the nail is left long enough to clear the underlying skin of the top of the toe and also be sure the edges of the nail do not penetrate the skin on the nail edge.

If you are unfortunate enough to get an ingrown toenail, you might consider consulting a foot specialist to have it corrected. It is possible to treat an ingrown toenail yourself by soaking the afflicted toe in hot water three times a day until the nail and surrounding tissues are soft and pliable. Then lift the nail with a tweezers from the underlying skin and place a small piece of cotton underneath the nail to allow it to grow free. After it grows out, you can trim it properly.

Stress fracture

Stress or *fatigue fractures* of any of the bones of the foot are the result of continued or excessive pressures on the foot. They can be annoyingly painful, although not necessarily debilitating.

Soldiers whose foot anatomy cannot withstand long marches have traditionally been the most frequent sufferers of stress fractures of one of the metatarsal bones of the foot. Now the most common sufferers of stress fractures are long-distance runners who train on hard surfaces like cement.

You may suspect that you are suffering from a stress fracture of the foot if you experience pain when running but little discomfort at other times, and also if the pain while running persists for more than two weeks, even at a reduced activity level. The surest way to diagnose a stress fracture is, of course, by X-ray examination.

The treatment of stress fractures is simple—rest. It is almost impossible to run or play through a stress fracture, although some athletes claim that they are able to do so by reducing their activity.

The prevention of stress fractures is not so simple. Although ideally, all one need do is eliminate the source of the stress (such as running on soft surfaces), that is not always possible. People who get involved in heavy training for running events or tennis matches sometimes must risk the occurrence of stress fracture in order to get into condition by working hard. Good sports shoes will offer some protection, as will attention to proper athletic form.

Fallen arches

The foot has two arches; one that bows the ball of the foot, and one that bows the inner side of the foot from front to back. Both arches are supported by ligaments in the foot.

A number of factors can cause the ligaments that support the arches to weaken and produce *fallen arches*. Overweight, faulty posture, ill-fitting shoes, and stress from overuse are some of the common ones.

83

Some people are born with "flat feet" and manage to get through life fairly well. But people who were born with normal arches and stress their foot ligaments to create fallen arches may experience pain and frequent foot fatigue. These people often need to place arch supports in their shoes to help unstable ligaments heal, while at the same time they need to correct whatever bad habit causes the problem. Usually that means tossing out an old, well-worn pair of sports shoes. Often hydrotherapy given in a whirlpool bath and rehabilitation exercises will help as well.

Heel bruise

Dancers, hurdlers, and basketball players are frequently subject to *heel bruise*—a forceful compression of the heel, usually caused by landing on the heel after a jump. Heel bruises (also known as stone bruises) can be very painful and therefore incapacitating for several days.

The treatment of heel bruises is like that of other contusions—ice, compression, and elevation immediately after the injury followed by heat treatments until the pain goes away. It is also wise not to put pressure on the heel for the first day or so of healing lest the trauma be aggravated.

Because heel bruises often arise as a consequence of a particular routine athletic activity, a person may experience them with some regularity. To protect yourself from heel bruises, either wrap the heel with protective tape, cushion the heel with moleskin, or buy a plastic heel cup to be inserted into the sports shoe.

Ankle Problems

The ankle is a joint comprised of the *tibia* bone of the lower leg and the *talus* of the foot. These bones form a *mortice-and-tenon* joint of considerable strength, and the entire ankle region is supported by several ligaments. The architecture of the ankle, however, allows primarily a hinge-like motion of the foot relative to the lower leg; therefore, the joint is vulnerable to strong forces exerted from the side.

84

Ankle sprain is one of the most common sports injuries, if not the commonest. The ankle is constructed to permit flexion and extension, but it is not constructed to withstand strong forces from the side that often accompany the twisting and jumping involved in athletics. If forces from the side are very strong, the ligaments that support the ankle can be stretched, partially torn, or even completely ruptured, resulting in a sprained ankle.

Several ligaments attach the leg bones to the bones of the foot. The function of these ligaments is to stabilize the ankle joint so that the bones do not move to the side when the foot is in motion. The ligament on the medial (inner) side of the foot is called the *deltoid ligament*. It fans out from an attachment on the *medial malleolus* (the knobby, protruding bone on the inner side of the ankle) to the bones of the foot. The lateral aspect (outside) of the ankle is supported by the *lateral ligaments,* which fan out from the *lateral malleolus* to the talus and calcaneus. The lateral ligaments resist inversion movement.

As strong as these ligaments are, they are not made of steel, and their fibers can be wrenched apart by extraordinary forces.

The symptoms of sprained ankle are pain, swelling, and a relative loss of function depending on the number of ligament fibers that have been damaged. Mild sprains, in which there is some pain but no loss of function, can heal within a few days with rest. Moderate to severe sprains, in which there is a great deal of swelling and total or almost total loss of function, require more care. The ankle should be immobilized for six to eight weeks to allow the repair of the ligaments. Even if the pain has subsided and the injury feels fine, the ligaments may nevertheless be weak if the necessary period for repair has not been alotted. By renewing activity too soon, you only increase the chance of doing permanent damage.

The ankle is a relatively strong joint and therefore not easily injured. However, there are things one can do to help prevent ankle injury. Strengthening the muscles of the lower leg offers perhaps the best preventive measures (see chapter 6). You can wear high-top sports shoes, as do many professional athletes, to give the ankle additional support. And if you are planning to jog along a country road or play softball in a city park, it would be wise to keep an eye out for ruts, gopher holes, and sprinkler systems.

9 Leg Problems

Lower Leg

The principal functions of the lower leg are movement of the foot about the ankle joint and transmission of the body weight to the ground. That is, not only are the bones and muscles of the leg organized to produce motion, but they are also aligned to support the entire weight of the body while still maintaining flexibility and balance.

The lower leg consists of two bones: the *tibia* on the inner aspect (big toe side) of the leg, and the *fibula* on the outer aspect (little toe side) of the leg. These bones are connected to each other along their adjacent sides by a fibrous membrane. The tibia is larger than the fibula and it alone is attached to both the knee and ankle. In other words, the tibia is, as the song goes, the "leg bone connected to the ankle bone."

The lower ends of the tibia and fibula have rounded projections called *malleoli,* which are easily felt as the bony protuberances of the ankle.

The principal actions of the muscles of the lower leg involve moving the foot at the ankle joint. Lifting the heel is called *plantar flexion*. (The sole of the foot is its plantar surface.) This movement is accomplished by contraction of the calf muscles. Lifting the top part of the foot toward the leg is called *dorsiflexion*. (The top of the foot is the dorsal surface.) Contraction of the muscles in the front of the lower leg produces dorsiflexion. Many of the muscles on the lateral part of the leg turn the sole of the foot outward (called *eversion*), and muscles on the medial side of the leg turn the sole inward (called *inversion*).

LOWER LEG CONTUSIONS

Lower leg contusions (bruises) very commonly are incurred by soccer players, who are particularly vulnerable and sensitive to being kicked, bumped, hit, and battered. That is because there is so little fat and muscle in that part of the leg to absorb shocks and bumps. Whenever the front of the lower leg receives a forceful blow, the result is compression damage to the skin and underlying tissues, the consequence being leakage of fluid and blood in the site of the injury. This causes swelling, pain, and sometimes loss of function. Often a blood clot will form in the injury site and the skin will become black-and-blue.

Although it does not happen often, sometimes a contusion in the front of the leg can present a serious medical problem. Because the structures in the front of the leg are enclosed in a fairly tight space between the skin and the tibia, any swelling from a contusion cannot expand very much, and the buildup of fluid pressure inside the leg can compress leg arteries and cut off blood to the muscles, resulting in their destruction.

The possibility of serious complications from injuries to the front of the leg makes trainers and team physicians watchful of the progress of the healing of bruises and soreness in that region. If within two weeks from the time of injury the inflammation and pain persist, intensive medical management may be necessary.

A blow to the back of the leg may be less serious than one to the front, but it is no less painful. Getting kicked in the calf can really hurt and can put the leg out of commission for several days.

If all you get in a struggle for a rebound is a kick in the calf, or if your squash opponent hits a low screaming shot that cracks you in the back of the leg, the best thing you can do is to apply I.C.E.

immediately and perhaps gently stretch your injured leg muscle. In a day or two, after you are sure the hemorrhaging has stopped, you can facilitate healing by applying heat treatments, and taking warm-water baths or whirlpool treatments. Massage and mild stretching are also beneficial.

Wearing protective padding is a good way to minimize the damage and disability from contusions. Soccer, field hockey, and rugby players often wear pads tucked inside their knee socks to absorb some of the blows. And without shin guards a baseball catcher or home plate umpire is out of uniform. The only padding available for the back of the legs that will not hamper movement is thick stockings.

Shin splints is an all-too-familiar ailment for track athletes, tennis players, and basketball players. Those who play volleyball occasionally suffer shin splints too.

The exact cause of shin splints is still debated by sports-medicine people. On the other hand, there is almost universal agreement among athletes about how shin splints feel: tenderness and pain along the entire inner front of the lower leg, extending from just below the knee all the way to the ankle.

Most experts agree that shin splints are the result of inflammation of the tendon of the posterior tibialis muscle or the interosseous membrane that connects the tibia and fibula. What they cannot agree on is what causes the inflammation. The suggestions include faulty posture, falling arches, muscle fatigue, overuse stress, body-chemical imbalance, and lack of proper reciprocal muscle coordination.

The recommended treatment for shin splints is a few days of rest and heat treatments, either from a heating pad or whirlpool bath. There is some disagreement as to whether supportive taping or wrapping or padding is of any help. Some athletes simply run through their shin splints, which, of course, is only possible if the pain is not too great. If an athlete with shin splints cannot rest, two aspirin and a ten-minute ice packing before working out or competing might help.

The best treatment for shin splints, of course, is prevention. Do not overuse the leg muscles—especially when active on hard surfaces. Wear good supportive shoes and build up the activity time gradually so that the legs can work into shape. If possible, begin training on soft surfaces like grass until the legs are strong enough to withstand the trauma from running on cement or jumping on a gymnasium floor. If you suspect that faulty foot or arch anatomy is causing your shin splints, a foot specialist who is knowledgeable about sports can probably design corrective inserts for your athletic shoes.

Muscle cramps come in two forms: *clonic spasm,* in which there is intermittent contraction and relaxation, and *tonic spasm,* in which the muscle is in constant contraction. Either way, they are painful and extremely distressing.

The best thing to do when someone gets a cramp is to relax the contracted muscle and the afflicted person as well. Firmly grasp the affected muscle and gradually stretch it until the cramp is relieved. Gentle massage may then be helpful. Some muscle cramps are caused by a lack of oxygen in the muscle and relief can be achieved by deep breathing, which may relax the person as well as relieve the cramps.

It is generally thought that most cramps are caused by excessive loss of body fluid and/or minerals through perspiration, or muscle fatigue. One way to help prevent cramping, therefore, is to replace fluids and minerals when perspiring heavily. Several fortified liquids (Sportade, Gatorade, and other drinks) that are designed to replace lost body salts are commercially available. Orange juice spiked with potassium, magnesium, and calcium salts may be a good homemade salt-replacing drink.

If there has been a lot of sweating, an extended period of rest and fluid replacement is best before returning to competition.

TENDON INJURIES

The tendons of the leg muscles that control movements of the foot are particularly vulnerable because the ankle joint is so active in sports. Tendon injury can involve either strain (overstretch) of a tendon or complete rupture. The former will cause pain and relative loss of function, whereas the latter will cause not only pain, but also

89

severe swelling and complete loss of function. Repeated overstress of any tendon can lead to chronic inflammation of the tendon, called *tendinitis,* or its surrounding sheath, called *tenosynovitis*. These are painful conditions that may take weeks or even months to heal.

Common tendon injury sites in the leg are the *Achilles tendon,* which attaches the calf muscles that control plantar flexion to the heel bone; the tendon of the *anterior tibialis muscle,* which controls dorsiflexion and inversion of the foot; the tendons of the *peroneal muscles,* which control eversion of the foot; and the *plantaris tendon,* a long thin tendon involved in plantar flexion.

Rupture of the Archilles tendon can occur if an enormous pull is exerted on the tendon, such as pushing off with the forefoot when the knee is locked and the lower leg extended. Another cause of Achilles tendon rupture is receiving a blow in the area of the tendon when the heel is lifted. This places a strong stretching force on the tendon when it is already taut.

When the Achilles tendon ruptures, a person may feel a sudden snap or feel as if someone has clobbered the back of the leg with a stick. There is severe pain all around the lower leg but particularly near the point of rupture. Swelling and discoloration from the leaking of fluid into the injured area occur quite soon after the initial trauma. And the person cannot lift the heel.

The swelling should be brought under control by I.C.E., and medical attention should be sought immediately. The preferred treatment of Achilles tendon strain is complete immobilization of the leg in a cast for about eight weeks, with the heel raised slightly to allow the tendon fibers to knit. Depending on the severity of the injury, surgical repair of the tendon may be necessary.

The plantaris muscle arises from the femur and passes under the gastrocnemius (the bulgy calf muscle) to attach to the Achilles tendon or middle part of the calcaneus. The belly of the muscle is only about two to four inches long, but the tendon is very long and thin, like a piece of twine.

Because the plantaris tendon is so thin it can easily be ruptured. When this happens one feels a burning pain deep in the calf. But because the plantaris is small, there is little loss of function. It is still possible to lift the heel, although there may be a great deal of accompanying pain.

90

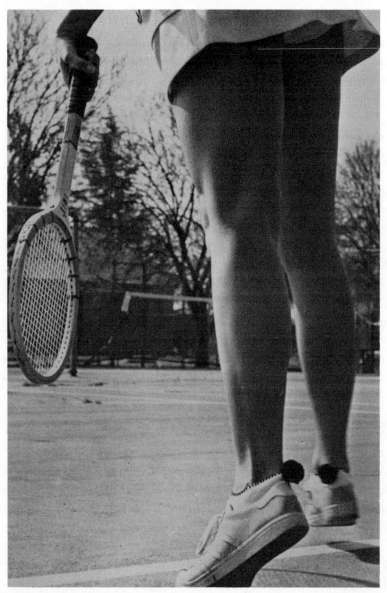

Tendons in the lower leg.

It is unlikely that an immobilizing cast will be necessary to treat a plantaris tendon injury, but a period of rest and perhaps bandaging for about six to eight weeks will be needed to allow the tendon to heal.

The problem with a plantaris tendon injury (as with almost any injury) is that while healing takes place, the injured person must discontinue all sports activity, and so gets out-of-shape. Moreover, if the leg is bandaged, the muscles become weak from disuse. Therefore, it is imperative that the leg muscles be strengthened before returning to activity. Otherwise the plantaris tendon may become injured again, or worse, damage may result to the Achilles tendon.

The peroneal muscles extend along the outside (lateral side) of the leg and insert on the foot to effect eversion of the foot. These are two major peroneal muscles, the *long peroneal* muscle and the *short peroneal* muscle. They each send tendons through a groove along the back edge of the lateral malleolus, the knobby part of the ankle. Powerful blows to the side of the ankle can sometimes pop the tendons out of their groove. Then surgery is required to replace them. More commonly, the tendons become inflamed from overuse, and tendinitis results.

Treatment of peroneal tendinitis is the same as for any other tendon: rest, mild stretching, and therapeutic heat treatments.

Upper Leg

The upper leg consists of a single bone called the *femur*, the largest in the body, which connects the hip and the knee. Collectively, the muscles in the front of the upper leg are called the *quadriceps group* (there are four of them), and their function is to straighten the leg—also referred to as extending the knee. Bending the leg or flexing the knee is the function of a group of muscles in the back of the thigh, collectively called the hamstrings.

Perhaps the most common injury to the quadriceps muscles is contusion from various kinds of direct blows, such as being hit with a hockey stick, other player's knees, wild pitches, and occasionally an errant elbow. The resulting contusion, called a *charley horse,* can be alarmingly large, extremely painful, and hideously ugly. Soon after the injury walking may be difficult at best, and it may take well over a week to recover, even with the aid of heat and massage therapy.

The hamstring group of muscles in the back of the thigh is subject to strains more often than contusions. These muscles are strained most commonly in sports that involve sprinting or fast starting movements like basketball, football, and various track and field events.

A hamstring pull is very painful, feeling somewhat like getting walloped in the back of the leg with a baseball bat. Sometimes the injured athlete can feel the muscle fibers tear at the moment of injury—just before he or she begins to limp.

A hamstring pull should be treated immediately with I.C.E., and then heat and gentle massage for the duration of the healing period, which usually is several days, although it can take weeks in the most severe cases.

10 Knee Problems

There is a famous photograph of Joe Namath sitting half-dressed in his football uniform in a locker room after a professional football game. There is the look of fatigue and pain on his face; he has played hard. And that is all the more amazing considering the state of his knees—they are constricted by layers of tape and smothered with straps and braces. It is a wonder he can walk—let alone play football.

This photograph is testimony to one of the best-known truisms about professional sports, namely, that knee injuries have hampered and prematurely ended more professional sports careers than any other injury.

The problem is that the knee is a vital joint but it lacks sufficient internal strength to withstand the twists, turns, and stresses involved in most sports activity. Football presents the greatest risk to knees, but basketball, baseball, skiing, and tennis take their toll as well.

Structure of the Knee

The function of the knee is to bend. Its allowable motions are flexion and extension. A small degree of rotation is also possible, but that is not the knee's principal movement.

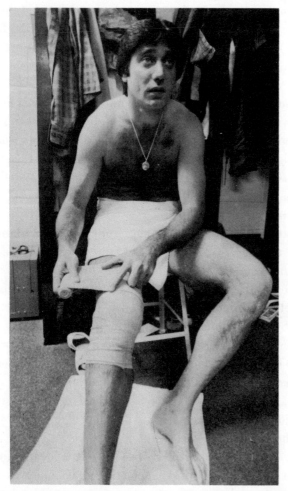

Joe Namath readies his knees for the stress of football.
UPI Photo.

Knee flexion and extension are controlled by the muscles of the thigh. There are four extensor muscles in the front of the thigh, collectively called the quadriceps. They originate on the femur, the thigh bone, and extend to the lower leg. When they contract they pull the foreleg up to straighten the leg. The hamstring group, a collection of seven muscles located in the back of the thigh, are the knee flexors. Some members of the hamstring group originate on the hip and others on the femur. They extend to the back of the lower leg so that when they contract, they cause the leg to bend at the knee.

The knee joint itself is comprised of three bones—the femur, or thigh bone (the largest bone in the body); the tibia, or shin bone; and a small triangular-shaped bone called the *patella*. The patella is the kneecap.

The femur has two rounded protuberances at its lower end called *femoral condyles*. The condyles fit into slight depressions in the tibia. Seated on the tibia are two oval disks (like rubber washers) of tough cartilage called *menisci*. There is a *medial meniscus* and a *lateral meniscus*. The menisci function to allow rotation of the femur on the tibia. Injured menisci are the "torn cartilages" so often mentioned in relation to knee injuries.

The patella or kneecap is situated in front of the articulation of the femur and tibia. The patella is held in place by tendons and ligaments that connect it to the femur and the tibia.

The bones of the knee joint are held in place by a remarkably complex set of ligaments and tendons. The front of the knee is supported by the tendon of the quadriceps muscles; the sides by ligaments called *collateral ligaments*—the *medial collateral* ligament on the inside of the leg and the *lateral collateral* ligament on the outside. The collateral ligaments help support the knee by prohibiting side-to-side movements. The lateral side of the knee is supported by an additional set of ligaments, and the back of the knee by a group known as the posterior ligaments.

The knee is further stabilized by two ligaments located inside the joint. These ligaments crisscross each other and hence are called the *cruciate ligaments*. The *anterior cruciate* ligament extends from the tibia to the lateral part of the femur and the posterior *cruciate* ligament extends from the tibia to the medial part of the femur. The function of the cruciate ligaments is to prevent the femur from slipping forward or backward on the tibia.

The entire knee joint is surrounded by an extensive synovial membrane that lubricates the joint. The membrane surrounding the knee forms many pockets known as bursa, any of which can become inflamed enough to cause bursitis in the knee.

Knee Injuries

By far the largest number of injuries to the knee are sprains—tears and associated damage to the ligaments that support the joint.

There are two reasons for this. First, the knee is inherently weak. The femur and tibia do not interconnect in any stable way, therefore, the integrity of the knee joint depends entirely on the supporting ligaments and tendons. The second, and probably the most important reason, is that many sports movements require sudden changes in body direction with the foot planted firmly on the ground and the knee extended, such as the cut-back in football or tennis. This movement can exert tremendous lateral forces on the knee, and if they are strong enough to overcome the tensile strength of the knee ligaments and tendons, the knee will collapse.

Perhaps the most common type of knee sprain involves damage to the medial side of the knee caused by a strong force from the side pushing the knee inward. In such cases fibers in the medial collateral ligament tear and perhaps even the entire ligament ruptures. If the force is severe enough, there can be additional

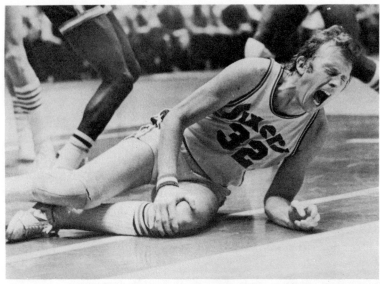

Billy Cunningham's knee injury ended his playing career. *UPI photo.*

97

damage to the medial meniscus, since it is attached to the medial collateral ligament. And if that is not enough, still further damage is possible to the anterior cruciate ligament, resulting in what is bemoaningly referred to in sports medicine as the "unhappy triad."

Virtually all the knee ligaments are vulnerable to injury. Any can be damaged by severe knee rotations or strong jolts from falling down or getting kicked in the knee. That is why football players and basketball players often wear knee pads.

The treatment of knee sprains depends on their severity. Mild sprains may require only a day or two of rest and then gradual return to activity. More severe sprains may require a longer period of rest to allow the ligament fibers time to repair. Some doctors elect to tape the leg heavily or immobilize it in a cast to be sure the repair process can proceed unimpeded by movement. In the most severe knee sprains, particularly those involving damage to the menisci (cartilages), surgery may be required to repair ligaments, tendons, and to remove pieces of menisci that may have been crushed in the injury.

Patellar injuries occur because of the patella's exposed position in the front of the knee. It has no overlying fat or muscle to protect it from injury in falls or receiving blows. It is right out there to take the lumps.

Severe stress can cause dislocation of the patella, in which case the quadriceps tendon, enclosing the patella, moves from its normal position in front of the knee to the side, usually over the lateral condyle of the femur. Severe blows can also cause fracture of the patella.

A patellar injury that basketball and volleyball players sometimes sustain is "jumper's knee," which is known medically as *patellar tendinitis*. This malady is caused by overuse of the patellar tendon from jumping vertically, such as rebounding in basketball or spiking in volleyball. The rapid flexion-to-extension movement that produces vertical jumping puts considerable strain on the tendon, and if the quadriceps is weak, inflammation in the form of tendinitis will result. The normal treatment of patellar tendinitis is rest and heat therapy.

The most effective ways to avoid patellar tendinitis are to

strengthen the quadriceps muscles with specific conditioning exercises—like the knee extension exercise and stair run described in chapter 6, and to avoid constant jumping movements that may bring on the injury.

Another patellar injury involves a degenerative process in which the patella softens and wears away. This condition is called *chondromalacia patellae*. People suffering from this condition experience pain, swelling, and sometimes a locking sensation in the knee.

Often chondromalacia patellae occurs after some other knee injury. Any problem that impedes the smooth movement of the patella can result in the wearing away of the underside of that bone as it rubs against one of the femoral condyles.

Chondromalacia patellae requires professional management that includes specific exercises to strengthen the quadriceps muscles; in some cases the use of antiinflammatory drugs like cortisone, and in the most severe cases, corrective surgery. Not attending to this condition can lead to gross degeneration of the patella and part of the femoral condyle, and hasten the onset of arthritis.

Bursitis is caused by continuous bruising of the knee and is characterized by inflammation in one of the many bursae of the knee region. The irritation will produce an excess of the synovial fluid that fills the bursal sac, sometimes producing pain but rarely loss of function.

Some team doctors simply drain an enlarged bursa with a needle. Others recommend protective padding and compression, and, of course, time to allow the swelling to regress, as a treatment.

Water on the knee is caused by traumatic injury to the knee that produces an accumulation of fluid in the joint. The fluid is not water, bur rather synovial fluid—the lubricating substance of joints, which is being produced in excess because of inflammation of the knee caused by the trauma.

Water on the knee is not an isolated knee problem, but a symptom of some other knee ailment. The treatment of water on the knee, therefore, is to correct the causative problem. Doctors sometimes aspirate (drain) the knee with a needle to relieve the discomfort from the accumulation of the extra fluid.

11 Back, Hip, and Pelvic Problems

Many jocks have back and hip problems. One reason for this is that we walk in the upright position. Because we stand erect, our back and hip muscles have to support the entire upper body against the pull of gravity, but because our animal ancestors walked around on all fours, our back and hip architecture has not evolved the necessary anatomical features needed to provide us with a strong back. Therefore, the back and hip are inherently vulnerable to injury, especially when you consider all the twisting, bending, and throwing motions involved in sports activity.

Anatomy of the Back

The back consists of the spinal column and numerous muscles and ligaments that hold the spinal column together and attach it in place to the shoulder and pelvis. There are over 400 muscles in the back.

The spinal column itself has thirty-three bones. These are the *vertebrae*. Twenty-four of the vertebrae are moveable and they provide the spine the flexibility to bend and twist. They are the upper vertebrae and extend from the neck to the lower back. The lowest five of these are the *lumbar vertebrae*, which are the largest and most moveable of the vertebrae. The lowest nine vertebrae are immoveable; they are fused to form the *sacrum* and *coccyx,* the tail bone.

The vertebrae are separated by *intervertebral disks*—small washer-like structures that separate the vertebrae from one another. Each intervertebral joint contains one intervertebral disk. The disks act as shock absorbers and also allow the vertebrae to move easily.

Back Injuries

Back injuries can be very serious, and in all cases a back specialist should be consulted if back problems arise.

Many back problems are caused by anomalies in the structure of the spine that are present from birth but only become noticeable when a person develops a back problem from sports activity. Usually, the problem takes the form of a sharp pain either in the lower back, under the shoulder blades, or between them. The pain can be so severe that walking and certain arm movements are almost impossible. The underlying problem is most likely a muscle strain in one or more of the many muscles in the back caused by an unusual twisting motion or perhaps running when off balance. The only solution to this kind of problem is to rest and apply heat treatments and massage to speed recovery. Increasing body flexibility may help prevent future injuries, and improving one's posture may also help.

Lower back pain is the bane of many an athlete's existence. "Oh my aching back" is the hackneyed phrase that often accompanies lower back pain, probably the most common medical complaint both on and off the athletic field. Television ads for low back-pain remedies are almost as frequent as those for toothpaste.

Several terms are often used interchangeably to describe this condition. *Sciatica, lumbosacral sprain,* and *sacroiliac sprain* are probably the most frequently mentioned. Each of those terms identifies a different part of the anatomy of the lower back and pelvic area.

The incidence of lower back pain increases with age. That is because many lower back conditions arise only after years of minor stresses from activity with an anatomically weak back, and also because as people get older their abdominal muscles lose tone and strength, and greater demands are placed on the back muscles and ligaments to support the upper torso.

101

If you suffer from chronic low back pain, the remedy to your problem lies in getting proper supervision from a specialist to strengthen the muscles in the pelvic and back region to take the strain off already weak and painful structures. If your back pain is related to a specific sports injury, it is best to have medical help to aid repair and rehabilitation of the injury.

Herniated (ruptured) disk is a condition that has ruined many a football career. It is the result of sudden blows to the back that exert so much pressure on one of the intervertebral disks that it cracks, and the soft gelatinous shock-absorbing material inside the disk leaks out. This material may place pressure on some of the spinal cord nerves and cause extreme pain. The only treatment is surgical repair of the disk followed by rehabilitation of the back to restore flexibility.

Hip Problems

The hip joint is formed by the articulation of the large bone of the thigh (the femur), and the bony pelvis through a ball-and-socket joint. The top of the femur is rounded, and that "ball" fits into a depression, the "socket" of the pelvis. Several strong ligaments support the hip joint so well that it is considered to be the strongest joint in the body. Hence, it is not injured very often, although muscle strains and ligament injury do occasionally occurr when a person twists with unusual force or falls down in a contorted position.

The treatment of hip muscle or ligament injury is the same as for any other similar injury; I.C.E. at first, followed by rest and gradual return to activity.

Football and hockey players wear hip pads to protect themselves from the "hip pointer." This is a bruise of the hipbone referred to in medical language as the *iliac crest*. It is the bony part of your side. The fact that you can feel the iliac crest is precisely why it is subject to bruising; it is right out there exposed to kicks, blocks, and hitting the ground or ice when one falls. These traumas mash the soft tissue overlying the bony iliac crest. The result is a very painful bruise that aches deep into the bone. So bad is the pain that it may be impossible to bend or even walk.

Naturally, cold and pressure should be applied immediately after a person suffers a hip pointer, and later, rest and heat treatments to speed recovery, which takes about two weeks.

The best way to prevent a hip pointer is to wear protective padding over the iliac crest and perhaps support it additionally with tape.

Pelvic Problems

A bone in the pelvic region that sometimes is injured when one receives a direct blow is the coccyx. The coccyx is the lower part of the spinal column, and you can feel it as the hard bony place between your thighs. Injuries to the coccyx usually occur with forced sitting down, such as taking a fall when you are ice skating or roller skating. Since the coccyx is a bony structure, persistent pain from that region should signal the need for medical attention to check for dislocation or fracture.

Groin strain is a sometimes incapacitating injury that can tend to recur with certain athletes. The groin is the region of the body at the top of the thigh and just below the abdominal area, anatomically termed the *inguinal region*. Some people mistakenly believe that the groin is a euphemism for the male genital region, but it is not. Women have groins too.

Several muscles traverse the groin as they extend from the pelvic bone to the thigh bone. A groin strain occurs when one or more of them becomes torn during strenuous activity.

A groin strain injury can produce a sudden twinge of pain the instant it happens, or it can sometimes not be noticed until activity stops. If groin strain is managed medically, it is likely that tests will be given to determine which muscle is hurt so that treatment can be applied directly to it.

The treatment for groin strain is rest and heat therapy. Sometimes supportive bandaging can help alleviate some of the pain and make walking and slow running possible.

A *hernia* is a medical term for the entry of some anatomical part of the body into another. Anything that bulges into another space is

103

said to *herniate*. In most cases a hernia involves the protrusion of some part of the internal organs of the abdomen through the abdominal muscles to the area just below the skin.

In men, the most common site of hernia is in the groin. This is the so-called inguinal hernia. Extreme abdominal pressure, such as when straining to lift something or straining during some violent activity can force a part of the intestinal organs through a natural space between the overlying pelvic muscles. The result is a painful injury treatable only by surgical repair.

A *scrotum contusion*, as one who has ever received one knows, is an agonizingly painful injury and when it happens to someone else there is nervous laughter among the men who have been spared. The injury involves getting hit or kicked in the scrotum, and so excruciating is the pain that the man doubles over and cannot do anything but groan.

Fortunately, there are two methods to relieve the immediate discomfort of a scrotal contusion. One is to lie the injured man on his back and flex his thighs to his chest. If possible, he can try to breathe deeply to try to relieve the muscle spasms in the testicular region.

A second technique involves having the injured man sit with his legs extended and his arms crossed on his chest. Someone stands behind him and lifts him by his folded arms a couple of inches off the ground and then drops him. Although this may seem like further torture, it turns out that the mild shock often releases painful muscle spasms.

Menstrual problems are usually dealt with effectively by most women. A problem can arise, however, in knowing how to integrate menstruation with athletic activity.

Many women can remember the times in their adolescence when they were prohibited from playing sports in gym class because they were menstruating. Fortunately, the faulty logic of that prohibition has been forgotten and been replaced by the dictum that a woman should do what feels comfortable for her. There is no reason why a woman cannot run, swim, or play tennis during her period if she feels OK about it.

If she suffers from severe cramps, she may not feel like doing anything, and that is her choice.

Many college and professional women athletes who experience menstrual difficulties take birth control pills both to relieve some of their menstrual discomforts (one of the few beneficial side effects of the pill) and also to regulate their periods in order to avoid menstruating during the time of an important competition.

Stitch-in-the-side, or side ache, is an incredibly painful cramping sensation in the upper part of the abdomen that occurs during a hard run. It can happen on either the left or right side and feels as if a hot, smoldering coal about the size of a baseball has been put in your side.

The most common cause of a stitch is cramping of the *diaphragm,* the muscle in the chest that effects breathing. When the diaphragm is called upon to do a lot of unaccustomed work to produce rapid and deep breathing because you are running hard it may cramp from fatigue—just as a leg muscle might cramp under similar overwork conditions. Stitch might also involve cramping of the muscles that join the lower ribs, for they are moving the rib cage up and down a lot during heavy breathing.

When stitch occurs the best thing to do is to relieve the cramp by stretching and deep breathing. To "stretch out" a stitch lift the arm on the affected side over the head as high as possible and stretch the muscles on that side of the body. Another helpful stretch is to bend forward at the waist and stretch the arms over the head. Taking deep breaths helps, too, because lack of oxygen is usually one of the problems.

Usually stitch occurs when a person is running hard to get back into shape after a layoff. Once the body is conditioned to hard running stitches should be few and infrequent. If for some reason they tend to persist even when the body is in shape, it may be time to consult a specialist. Sometimes stitch is caused by faulty breathing technique while running, and a coach or trainer may be able to offer guidance on how to correct this.

Persistant pain in the upper right part of the abdomen may indicate a dietary cause of stitch. In this instance stitch is the result of gas accumulating in the transverse colon and distending that organ to the point that it causes pain. One suggested treatment for stitch is to refrain from eating for six to twelve hours before running.

105

Another remedy is to eat foods that contribute to bulk in the gastrointestinal tract, such as fruits and vegetables. Diets high in protein and starch (potatoes, spaghetti and certain other food) apparently contribute to the trapping of gas in the colon, which aggravates the occurrence of stitch.

12 Shoulder, Arm, and Hand Problems

Anthropologists theorize that one of the characteristics that contributed to the successful evolution of our species is the ability to use the hands. The shoulder evolved with an architecture that permits a nearly unlimited range of motion, and we possess the ability for the very finely coordinated movement of our hands and fingers. Unlike our primate ancestors, we walk upright so that our hands and arms do not share the responsibility of supporting the body weight and are free to throw and catch baseballs, hit backhands, shoot jumpshots, and spike volleyballs. Indeed, without our arms and hands, our sports activity would be relegated to variations of running and kicking sports. (Even running and "hand-less" sports such as soccer require some use of the arms and hands—for balance if for nothing else).

Anatomy

Considered as a whole, the upper limb consists of the shoulder, upper arm, forearm, wrist, and hand. Excluding the movements of the fingers, the motions of the upper limb occur at the shoulder joint, the elbow joint, and the wrist joint.

The shoulder is a ball-and-socket joint formed by the articulation of the rounded head of the bone of the upper arm, the humerus, and a depression in the triangular-shaped shoulder blade, the *scapula*. The joint is surrounded by a capsule of synovial membrane and contains several bursae. The entire structure is stabilized by several ligaments and the tendons of the muscles that effect the range of shoulder movements.

The elbow joint is made up of the humerus and the two bones of the forearm, the *ulna* and the *radius*. Unlike the shoulder, which can bend and rotate, the elbow is capable only of flexion and extension and a small degree of rotation.

The wrist is formed by the joining of the ends of the ulna and radius with three bones in the back of the hand. These attachments are stabilized by several ligaments and the tendons of the muscles located in the arm that control the movements of the wrist.

Most of the sports injuries that affect the upper limb are either fractures and dislocations of the shoulder and arm bones caused by falling or stress-induced inflammations of tendons from throwing and hitting balls. Injuries from falls are difficult to prevent, but stress injuries are relatively easy to avoid. The key is to strengthen the muscles involved and to throw or hit with proper form.

Shoulder Problems

Rough football play is a frequent cause of shoulder injuries. Blocking, tackling, and falling can cause muscle strains, fractures of the bones of the shoulder and the upper part of the humerus, and sprains and dislocations of the articulations that make up the shoulder joint.

The so-called separated shoulder is a dislocation of the articulation of the clavicle and scapula. It is usually caused by falling on the top of the shoulder or by breaking a fall by extending the arms. It is not unusual for someone to dislocate this joint repeatedly, for once the ligaments are stretched and torn in the first injury they may never regain their former strength.

Shoulder strain is often experienced by athletes who use a throwing motion in their sports (such as baseball pitchers, javelin throwers, and tennis players). They expose the muscle-tendon units of the upper arm and shoulder to overuse strain and the repurcussions of continual tendon strain—tendinitis and tenosynovitis.

The tendon of the biceps muscle of the upper arm is a frequent site of this kind of muscle-tendon unit irritation. The front of the upper arm aches and it becomes hard to move. There is likely to be point tenderness in the top front of the upper arm as well. What has happened is that the rotation motion from too much throwing or serving has irritated the tendon of the biceps at the attachment of the tendon to the scapula or, more commonly, the synovial membrane that surrounds the tendon becomes inflamed.

The treatment for shoulder tendinitis or shoulder tenosynovitis is complete rest for one or two weeks with daily heat treatments followed by special rehabilitation exercises for the shoulder to prevent recurrence. Shoulder exercises are presented in chapter 6.

Shoulder bursitis, an inflmmation of one or more of the bursae in the shoulder region, is another consequence of stress irritation in the shoulder. Remember that the function of bursae is to lubricate joints and their supporting structures, and stress inflammation of a particular region can induce a bursa to produce excessive fluid so that inflammation can be reduced. The excess fluid, however, does not relieve the irritation, but often produces pain and disability instead.

The principal treatment for shoulder bursitis is rest, and heat treatments to facilitate recovery. Occasionally, a doctor will drain the excess fluid from the affected bursa.

Arm Problems

Tennis elbow may be the most common sports injury in this country. It is difficult to find anyone around the courts who has not had a twinge of tennis elbow.

Tennis elbow is actually a grab-bag term for several specific pathological conditions, each of which produces a similar symptom: pain on the lateral (outside) part of the elbow that may be excruciating when gripping anything or twisting the wrist. The problem is that the tendons of the muscles involved in the extension (straightening) and outward rotation of the wrist pass over the *lateral epicondyle* of the humerus, which is the knobby lower part of that upper arm bone, and constant stress-irritation sets up an inflammatory response in that region. When the tendon of the *extensor-supinator muscles* of the forearm are directly involved, the condition is known as *lateral epicondylitis,* probably the most common form of tennis elbow.

The treatment of tennis elbow involves complete rest until the pain subsides and accompanying heat treatments. In severe cases surgery may be necessary. Some people receive cortisone injections to help reduce the inflammation, but this practice is questioned by some team doctors as being ineffectual and possibly harmful.

The key to preventing tennis elbow is strengthening the forearm muscles (try squeezing a rubber ball or tennis ball for thirty minutes a day) and perfecting a smooth and even forehand ground stroke. In fact, many tennis pros claim that the sole preventative measure for tennis elbow is proper form.

Wrist and Hand Problems

A *sprained wrist* is usually caused by the simple act of falling down. Putting your arms out in front of the body to break your fall tends to hyperextend the wrist and the impacting force damages the ligaments that support the joint.

A sprained wrist, like other ligament injuries, brings on swelling, pain, and some loss of function depending on the severity of the damage to the ligament fibers. The immediate treatment is I.C.E. Because many injuries to the wrist involve fracture of the *carpal navicular* bone of the wrist, it is wise to have an X-ray evaluation of any wrist injury to ascertain the extent of the damage. After a wrist sprain has been medically evaluated, treatment will involve a rest period to allow the ligament fibers time to repair and then an exercise program to strengthen the muscles of the forearm.

Finger problems such as fractures, dislocations, and tendon injuries are often experienced by baseball, basketball, and volleyball players. The cause of these injuries, of course, is getting hit with the ball. In all cases of injuries to the fingers or thumb, medical care should be sought to insure complete repair.

Baseball finger (also called mallet finger) is a permanently

110

deformed finger that results if proper treatment is not applied immediately. Baseball finger is produced when the ball strikes the tip of the finger so that the impact tears the extensor tendon away from the bone. This puts a thirty-degree bend in the end of the finger. Splinting and up to six weeks of rest are necessary for complete recovery.

13 Skin Problems

The skin bears the brunt of a lot of trauma during athletic activity. Some skin ailments even have sports-related names like "jock itch" and "athlete's foot." The rest are known by more general names such as cuts, scrapes, sunburn, and frostbite.

Of course, the skin's function is to protect us from many environmental hazards such as damaging sunlight, bacteria, and other infectious organisms. It also protects us from drying out and helps to maintain our internal body temperature at about ninety-eight degrees Fahrenheit. And through pain and the sense of touch the skin provides information about our environment. Nevertheless, the skin is not made of steel, nor are its nonliving proteinaceous appendages, the hair and nails, made of plastic. The skin is a living bilayered organ, and it is subject to damage by certain stresses.

Blisters are problems that every athlete knows about. They come free with the purchase of a new pair of athletic shoes. Tennis and racketball players are "fortunate" enough to know about blisters on the hand, too. Blisters are caused by friction. When the skin gets too hot from too much rubbing, a blister forms. Therefore, the best way to avoid blisters is to avoid exposing parts of the body to abnormal amounts of friction.

Blisters frequently occur on the feet when breaking in a new pair of shoes. It takes a while for your feet to find a way of matching their geometric needs within the limits imposed by machine-made shoes. While this process is going on it is possible to work up a blister on the heel, or side of the foot, or on the toes. Some people work up blisters on their feet along the seam of a shoe, and so they wear sports shoes with "unibody construction" in the front.

Some trainers recommend wearing two pairs of socks—a thin cotton sock underneath and a thick wool sock on top. If you choose to wear two pairs of socks, be sure you have your sports shoes fitted while wearing the socks. Also, be sure the socks fit snugly. If they are too big, they tend to wrinkle, which may cause blisters too.

Blisters on the racket hand usually occur because the grip on the racket is too big. Proper selection of equipment is the obvious solution for this problem. If the grip and the hand are properly matched and blisters are still a problem, one should attempt to toughen the affected skin by playing initially for short periods and then gradually increasing the playing time until the skin thickens or a callus forms. Some players try to avoid blisters on the racket hand by using a glove, or by taping the vulnerable region.

Blisters usually begin as "hot spots"—areas of the skin that get pink and tender from rubbing. Sometimes the skin of a hot spot is loose. If you develop a hot spot, or know that you are particularly vulnerable to blisters in a certain place, you should lubricate that area of skin with vaseline before you work out or play. You can also protect the area with Band-Aids, adhesive tape, or moleskin. In fact, some people carry vaseline, tape, and moleskin in their athletic bags just in case.

If you develop a blister, avoid the temptation to pick or pull at it. You might impede healing by exposing new skin before it is ready, or worse, you could easily contract an infection that has the potential to get into the bloodstream and cause serious trouble.

The best treatment for blisters is benign neglect. They will go away by themselves in a few days. If a blister is very large and you feel the need to drain it, use a sterile needle and poke gently under the skin near the blister to let out the water or blood. Do not puncture the blister or pull off the skin. As the blister heals and the overlying skin dries out, then its acceptable to cut off the dead skin.

Corns on the feet and *calluses* on the feet and on other parts of the body are other kinds of skin problems caused by friction, although in some specific cases, such as the racket hand of a tennis player, a callus might be beneficial. Corns and calluses on the feet, however, are almost never desirable.

The best way to handle corns and calluses is to prevent them. As with blisters, protect areas of the body that receive a lot of friction. This is done by wearing well-fitting shoes and other clothes, and using tape or moleskin to cover vulnerable areas.

If corns or calluses should occur, do not cut them off with a knife. Protect the regions with soft padding until they go away. If a corn or callus causes a great deal of trouble, go to a foot specialist for treatment.

Everybody knows what a scratch is. But do you know the difference between an *abrasion,* a *laceration,* and a *puncture?*

An abrasion is a scrape, like the one sustained from falling off a bicycle or sliding into second base. It is a reddened, rough sore that looks as if someone rubbed the skin with steel wool. In "jock" terminology, an abrasion is called a "strawberry." Baseball players protect themselves from getting strawberries by wearing sliding pads.

Lacerations and punctures are forceful breaks in the skin. The common name for a laceration is a cut, and a puncture is a hole produced by a sharp, pointed object like a nail.

The definition of these types of wounds is important when treating them. In all cases the object of treatment is to avoid infection and to facilitate healing without scarring. To avoid infection, it is mandatory that the wound be kept clean and therefore free of infectious organisms. To promote scar-less healing, the ends of the wound should be brought together and the body's normal healing process allowed to proceed. If a laceration is very large or if the edges are rough and jagged, it may be necessary to stitch the opposing edges together to be sure the wound knits properly.

Treating wounds is fairly simple. After they happen wash them out with warm water and a mild soap. In the case of abrasions this treatment is very important, since the surface that caused the abrasion could contain little sand particles, and pieces of glass and organic debris. Irrigate the region with warm (not hot!) water from a squirt bottle, or hold it under a tap, or swirl it around in a bucket or tub. If the injured area is bleeding slightly don't be alarmed. The person is not likely to lose a dangerous amount of blood, and the blood can help wash particles and bacteria out of the wound. When treating lacerations and punctures, use your common sense. You will certainly want to clean the wound but if there is a great deal of bleeding apply pressure over the wound to stop it first and then seek medical help to keep the wound closed and to help avoid infection. A beneficial treatment may be the application of tincture of iodine or antiseptic first aid creams. And if the injured person has not had a tetanus shot or tetanus booster within the previous two years, it might be wise to consult a physician.

Jock itch is a scaly rash that usually forms in the groin. It is a type of ringworm, which is caused by a fungus. Fungi are small micro-organisms that are related to plants. They thrive in warm, moist environments.

Jock itch is prevented by keeping the groin region clean and dry and never using anyone else's athletic clothes.

Treatment and control of jock itch is obtained through the use of powders and creams that contain *tolnaftate*. These powders and creams are available without prescription.

Athlete's foot is also a fungal infection. Most commonly, it starts in the toe-web space between the fourth and fifth toes. It may then spread to the rest of the foot.

Athlete's foot usually appears as a red, itchy scaly problem. Left untreated it may become painful and the skin may peel, blister, and even bleed. In this advanced stage a secondary bacterial infection may be involved and medical help should be sought. As with jock itch, athlete's foot fungus lives best in warm, wet environments, so care should be taken to keep the feet dry. Use clean cotton or wool socks so that air is more likely to circulate around the feet. Powdering between toes may also help. Give your athletic shoes a chance to dry out between uses. If you are prone to athlete's foot infections, perhaps two pairs of sports shoes is a good idea.

Basic treatment of athlete's foot involves the use of powders and creams that contain *tinactin*.

Sunburn is the result of exposing the skin to excessive amounts of ultraviolet radiation.

Avoiding sunburn is simple: protect the skin from overexposure to ultraviolet sunlight. The easiest way is to wear clothes—broad-brimmed hats, peaked caps, and tennis hats, for example. If you are a surfer or skier, you cannot wear a Panama hat when you are "doing your thing." Your best sunburn protection comes from creams and lotions that block the harmful light rays. Baby oil, quick tanning lotions, and cocoa butter are ineffective. The most effective lotions contain *para-aminobenzoic acid* (PABA) in alcohol and the best creams contain *cinnamates* and *benzophenones*.

It should be remembered that snow, sand, and water reflect ultraviolet rays and can, therefore, increase the dose of damaging radiation absorbed by the skin. Also remember that ultraviolet radiation can penetrate fog and clouds; therefore protective measures should be taken on overcast days as well as on sunny ones.

Frostbite occurs when the skin actually freezes. Small ice crystals form in the skin cells and destroy them. It most frequently occurs on the hands, feet, nose, and ears—any place where blood circulation is diminished as a result of exposure to cold.

Prevention of frostbite involves covering up and staying dry. If you run or play in very cold weather or cross-country ski, it is a good idea to check with others frequently to be sure your exposed skin surfaces are OK. If your skin gets white, cold, and painful, try to restore normalcy with the warmth from a hand or warm up very slowly with body-temperature water. Do not massage the skin too vigorously or use very hot temperatures to restore circulation. You might burn the skin.

Chafing is an annoying skin condition that affects athletes in many sports. It is caused by the rubbing of athletic clothes against skin wet with perspiration. The inner part of the thighs is probably the most frequently affected area, especially in distance runners, because their wet legs are constantly rubbing against their running shorts.

Probably the best way to prevent chafing is to apply vaseline or some other kind of grease to the vulnerable areas in order to lubricate the skin. Hand cream is not as effective as vaseline because it is water soluble and will tend to wash off. Women can avoid irritation from rubbing bra seams and fasteners if they pad their skin with a paper tape called *Dermacel*.

14 Injuries in Various Sports

All sports are not the same. Football is a team sport that involves a lot of body contact, whereas running and swimming are individual sports that require no body contact. The different demands made upon the body by participation in various sports makes certain injuries more likely in certain sports. Contusions, for example, are more likely in football than they are in running or swimming. What follows is a summary of the sports injuries that occur most commonly in various sports.

Basketball

Although you can't tell by watching college or professional level play, basketball is considered a noncontact sport. But high-level basketball players pay little attention to that fantasy. Close guarding, collisions with other players while running at nearly full speed, and aggressive rebounding all contribute to a host of different injuries. The most frequent injuries in basketball are broken fingers—usually incurred by jamming them against another player or the ball, and sprained ankles. Falling to the court floor while off-balance when rebounding is the cause of sprained ankles. Falling also causes skinned knees and elbows, bruises, and "strawberries" from skidding on the gym floor or outdoor court.

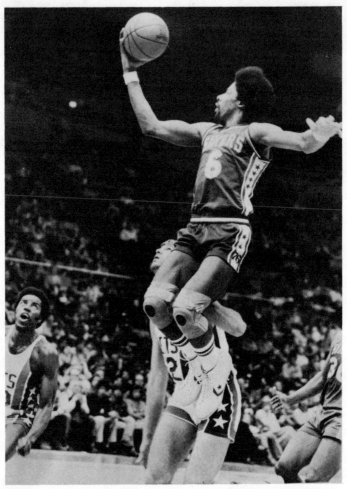

Dr. J. (Julius Erving) does all he can to protect his knees. *UPI photo.*

Those who play basketball a great deal risk certain injuries that are the bane of runners: patellar tendinitis, Achilles tendinitis, Achilles tendon rupture, and fatigue fractures of the bones of the feet.

Preventing injuries to the foot, ankle, and leg can be accomplished by strengthening the muscles in that region. The ankle-strengthening exercises presented in chapter 6 can help, as

118

can a daily routine of heel raises to improve jumping ability, and knee extension exercises to protect the knee. Foot and leg problems can also be avoided by wearing shoes that offer good arch support and have soles that cushion the many jars the feet suffer in each basketball game. Shoes with high tops or ankle taping can offer some protection against ankle sprain. Protective pads on the knees and elbows can help defend against scrapes from falling to the playing surface.

One additional injury-preventing scheme that seems to be all-important in college and professional basketball is a well-refereed game. Call 'em close!

Bowling

Bowling is a relatively mild sport. There is very little running and no contact with other players. Nevertheless, there are some ailments that bowlers should look out for. Sticking your tender fingers into that rock-hard ball and then using them as levers to hurl it toward the pins can be dangerous. Fingers can be bruised, dislocated, and even broken if they are pinched or trapped in the holes. Be sure that your ball fits your fingers well and your release is smooth.

Proper form in bowling is an essential for scoring well and also for staying injury-free. Hurling the ball while in a crouch or leaning to one side can wrench back, hip, and thigh muscles. Be sure to keep the back straight and bend the knees upon delivery. Also remember that throwing the ball very hard can strain the arm muscles, including the biceps and muscles of the shoulder. A regular routine of pushups can help strengthen the arm muscles to prevent throwing injuries. Another valuable exercise is the *pendulum*, (illustrated in chapter 6), a weight-swinging exercise seemingly designed for bowlers.

Cross-Country Skiing

Cross-country skiing is said to be the most physically demanding sport of all; it puts tremendous demands on the cardiorespiratory system (heart and lungs), so much so that cross-country skiers are arguably the best conditioned athletes. If you are just taking up the sport, as many are nowadays, and have any concerns at all about the condition of your heart or lungs, check with a specialist first.

Once on the snow, it is best to be concerned with protecting your exposed body regions. Clothes or antisunburn lotion that contains an effective sunscreen like PABA should cover the skin to protect from sunburn. Adequate clothing to protect the body from the cold should also be worn.

The feet are perhaps the most vulnerable part of your body to the ill effects of cold. They can be protected by waterproofing the boots and by wearing *gaiters,* special water-repellent boot coverings. Some people simply wear an extra pair of wool socks *outside* the boots.

Be sure to protect the eyes from sun and reflection damage with sunglasses or goggles. Excess ultraviolet radiation can damage the retina of the eye and impair vision.

To protect the legs from injury, one should be sure the leg muscles and tendons are stretched before beginning an outing. Be particularly mindful to stretch the Achilles tendons and the hamstrings as described in chapter 5.

When the terrain slopes downward the cross-country skier must beware of the types of hazards encountered by downhill skiers. Also be watchful for buried logs, rocks, and other hazards below the snow. Ski in groups so that if you are injured you will not have to face the cold alone while waiting to be helped.

Cycling

Cyclists must be aware of two types of injury—injuries sustained while actually riding and injuries from falling from the bicycle.

The most common riding injuries that affect cyclists are muscle cramps and small strains. These usually occur because the leg muscles are tired and/or the rider has perspired away needed water and minerals. Conditioning for long rides is perhaps the best way to prevent these kinds of injuries. By riding frequently, one will strengthen the leg muscles and also accustom the body to dealing with salt- and water-loss stress. If one is perspiring heavily attention

120

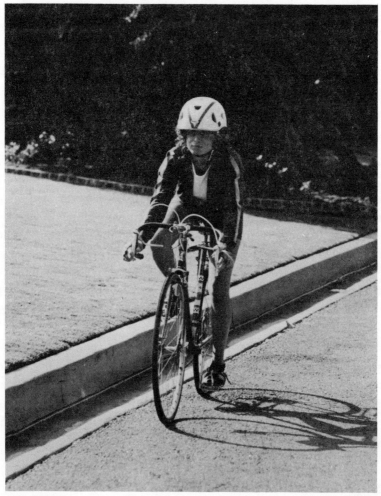

Cyclists have to protect their heads and hands in case of spills. *Photo by Barbara Bennett.*

should be paid to replacing water and minerals, particularly potassium, magnesium, and calcium. Some riders drink a glass or two of a fortified liquid like E.R.G. *before* they begin a race or workout to prevent muscle cramping from water and salt loss. They also carry replacement liquids with them.

121

Most cyclists are probably more concerned with collision injuries than muscle problems. Falling from the bicycle at reasonably high speed can be very dangerous, so cyclists try to protect themselves by wearing helmets, gloves, and elbow pads.

It is important to wear clean cycling clothes, too, for it is possible to get boils in the crotch from friction with the saddle.

Football

The best way to avoid injury in football is not to play the game at all. There are few sports in which the incidence of injury is as high as in football. Even with all their training, expertise, and protective equipment, professional and college football players sustain an enormous number of injuries. It is the nature of the game.

Even in a friendly touch football game, the occasional body contact leads to bruises, sprains, and sometimes even broken bones. The frequent changes in direction while running, being blocked, or falling down can wipe out a knee for life. And would-be quarterbacks can injure an arm or shoulder while throwing, which can cause weeks of pain.

If you must play football, be sure to rule out shoulder blocking, body blocking, and tackling as part of your game. Use your common sense and try to keep contact to a minimum. Use simple pass-blocking techniques and play "two-hand touch" instead of flag or tackle football. And give your knees and ankles a break by avoiding a lot of fancy footwork.

Golf

Proper form in the grip and swing can prevent many injuries common to once-a-week duffers. For example, relaxing the grip at the top of the swing may lead to an inflammation of the tendons of the thumb muscles, a condition that causes pain in the palm (right palm for left-handed golfers and left palm for right-handed golfers). The key to prevention is to tighten the grip when accelerating the club in the swing.

Golfers are also subject to strains in the muscles of the neck, shoulders, and back. Often these strains are the result of poor form, which leads to improper twisting in the swing. Consultation with a good golf teacher can help prevent these problems. Practicing flexibility exercises like the trunk-circling exercise and the abdominal twists (see chapter 6) can help.

Wrist and arm problems also hamper many a golfer. Tendinitis in the wrist can occur from increased cocking of the wrist on the backswing. And golfers who hold their club too tightly may suffer *lateral epicondylitis*—tennis elbow! To avoid these problems a golfer should use the wrist-and shoulder-strengthening exercises described in chapter 6.

Handball

Handball players are subject to all the common running and arm-swinging injuries that occur in racket sports. To avoid them be sure the legs and arms are loosened up before going onto the court, and try to give special attention to strengthening the ankle region with the heel-raise exercise and the shoulder with arm raises supplemented with weights.

Eye injuries are not infrequent in handball, and special eye guards, which are commercially available, should be worn.

As might be expected, hand injuries are also a problem to watch out for. Bone bruises can be avoided by warming the hands in hot water before play and wearing thin cotton gloves under the handball gloves.

Ice and Field Hockey/Lacrosse

These sports are rife with injuries to the face and body from getting hit with the stick or occasionally the puck or ball. Unfortunately, some coaches condone (and even encourage) body checking with the stick, which leads to many unnecessary bruises and lacerations.

The best protection against errant sticks and balls is to wear as much padding as possible. Ice hockey players do this routinely, but field hockey and lacrosse players don't wear padded uniforms as a rule, although lacrosse players wear protective headgear.

Because these sports involve a lot of leg motion, the common leg injuries (ankle sprain, knee sprain, muscle strain) prevail. One can try to prevent these injuries by building strength in the legs with the exercises for ankle, knee, and leg outlined in chapter 6.

Ice Skating

Ice skating injuries most often involve contusions and fractures that accompany falling down. There is not much you can do about that.

The condition of the ice that is skated upon can help prevent knee and ankle injuries incurred by catching the skate blades on flaws in the ice. Be sure to survey the ice you skate on to locate the dangerous spots.

You are asking for ankle trouble if you rent ice skates that are very old and offer little ankle support, or if they do not fit correctly. Be sure the skates fit snugly and that your ankle feels somewhat constrained.

Rugby

If you have ever seen a rugby game you will know why it is a game you play at your own risk—seemingly designed to see who can take the most punishment. Rugby players suffer a lot of contusions and abrasions. Some players wear protective padding in their knee socks and several layers of shirt under the rugby shirt to help absorb some of the blows and protect the skin from scrapes. Mouthguards are mandatory. In addition, some players apply vaseline to their faces to reduce the burn from friction during pile-ups.

Since rugby involves a lot of running and body contact, all foot, leg, knee, and shoulder injuries occur with some frequency. As with football, these injuries seem to be an inevitable part of the game, but strengthening all the body's muscles and being in good shape will obviously help.

Running

Running is one of the most strenuous athletic activities, and to

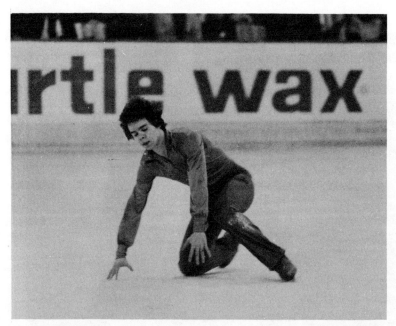

Ouch! *UPI photo.*

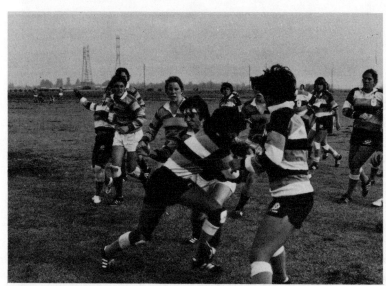

Rugby can be a brutal game. Play at your own (considerable) risk. *Photo by Crystal Chan.*

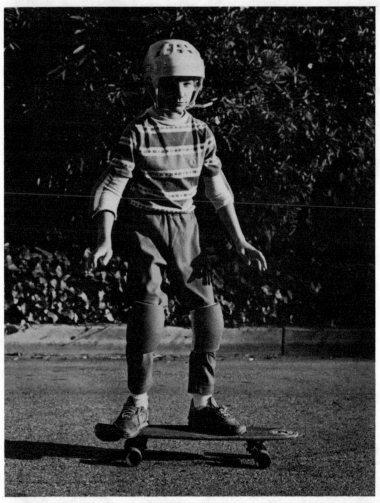

Stay off skateboards. Skateboard-related injuries are the most frequent in all amateur sports. *Photo by Barbara Bennett.*

avoid injury particular attention must be paid to the use of proper equipment (especially running shoes) and physical conditioning.

Without proper shoes and strong leg muscles, tendon and ligament injuries of the ankle, knee, and hip are almost inevitable. Be sure you are outfitted with shoes that fit properly and that offer good support. Work up to distances slowly so that your legs will build the strength needed to remain injury-free.

Particularly vulnerable body regions will, by being painful, make themselves known to anyone who runs. The wise runner will take heed and immediately embark on a training program designed to strengthen the complaining region. (See chapter 6).

Skiing

Skiing has the greatest ratio of leg injuries to other kinds of injuries. It also has one of the highest incidences of injury of any sport. Of the estimated five million skiers, it is estimated that about one million are hurt skiing each year.

About 50 percent of ski injuries are sprains of the ankle and knee, another 30 percent are the infamous skier's broken leg, and the others cuts and bruises. Very often the injury occurs when the skier catches the inside edge of one ski and the downhill momentum puts strong external rotational forces on the fixed leg. Improving strength in the muscles of the leg, particularly the quadriceps (to protect the knee), is the best way to avoid the more severe skiing injuries.

Since the incidence of ski injuries decreases in experienced skiers, form counts. Experience counts in another way too. Many novice skiers get hurt by trying to get the most action out of a single day's lift ticket and they push their body to the point of fatigue—a sure way to get hurt. Experienced skiers can sense when their body is tired and know it's time to quit.

When skiing, remember that snow reflects sunlight, so wear protective lotion to prevent sunburn, and sunglasses or goggles to protect the eyes.

Soccer

Due to the fact that soccer involves a lot of running and contact, soccer players suffer all types of leg muscle and ligament damage as well as such superficial injuries as abrasions, bruises, and sunburn. They also have to be careful of facial and eye injuries sustained from heading the ball.

Proper training to strengthen the leg muscles will help prevent leg injuries, and awareness of fatigue can help avoid muscle and tendon strains.

127

Softball

The smart softball player is cautious. Adequate warm-up before a game is necessary—especially for the throwing arm, the legs, and the back. If you are out of shape, it is probably wise not to run full speed in your picnic softball game. It may lead to pulled leg or back muscles. Run one-half to three-quarters speed instead.

Never slide into a base. Even if you were the stolen-base champion of your Little League, refrain from sliding. Too often the result is a torn-up ankle or knee that could cripple you for life. Professional ball players work long and hard on their sliding technique, and the ground upon which they slide is treated with that purpose in mind. It is unlikely, however, that the field in your local park is so treated.

Squash/Racquetball

The most common injuries in squash and racquetball are getting hit with the ball, the opponent's racquet, or the opponent. Ouch!

Blisters on the hand are sometimes a problem when first beginning regular play and can be avoided by graduated activity or by wearing protective taping or gloves.

Squash and racquetball players can suffer any of the leg injuries common to sports involving running. Good shoes and body flexibility can help keep ankle, leg, and knee problems to a minimum.

Tennis elbow is not a common problem in either of these court sports, but occasionally it happens. As with tennis, squash and racquetball require good form to improve performance and stay injury-free.

Surfing

Most surfing injuries come from the collision of the surfer with an errant surfboard. Such collisions cause their share of lacerations and broken bones.

Inexperienced surfers are vulnerable to getting hit by the board when they stand too far back on the tail, which risks having the board fly out from under them and bounce off the water. Surfers also get hurt when they bail out and the board comes down on top of them when they are in the water.

The best thing to do when you wipe out is to stay underwater as long as possible to let the board go its way. When you resurface put your hands over your head to protect the scalp and face. Some experienced surfers double up and bring their legs to their abdomen to protect their vital organs from injury from a wayward surfboard.

The well-known knee ailment called *surfers knots* is connective tissue growths on the knees that sometimes get as big as a golfball. Rest and no contact with a surfboard for a while is the best treatment.

Swimming

Swimming is a relatively safe sport. Apart from the usual overuse problems that can occur in any sport, swimmers are not particularly prone to any specific injury. Except for "swimmer's ear." Swimmer's ear is known medically as *external otitis*. It is an infection of the outer ear that is characterized by itching, drainage, tenderness, and sometimes a lot of pain. Treatment of this obnoxious disorder must be managed by a physician.

And yes, it is wise not to swim within an hour after eating. Competition for blood between the digestive system and the skeletal muscles can definitely lead to the onset of cramps.

Tennis

Since tennis involves a lot of running and quick changes in movement direction, injuries to the leg are most common in this sport. The best way to avoid them is by conditioning the leg to be strong and flexible and by warming up well before play. Also wear good supportive shoes.

The infamous tennis elbow problem is the result of an improper swing in combination with weak forearm muscles. If tennis elbow is to be avoided, one should perfect a smooth, flowing stroke, and try to avoid short, choppy, twisting strokes. Another possible preventative measure is to use lightweight aluminum rackets strung with gut. Do not be embarassed to walk around squeezing a tennis ball. Not only

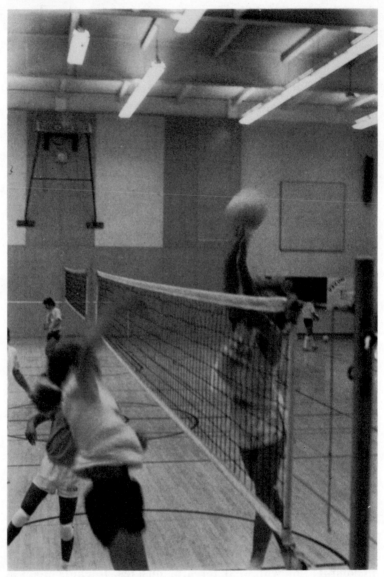

Look out for jammed fingers!

will it build strength in your forearm and help you be rid of tennis elbow, but it will also enhance your prestige as a serious athlete.

Volleyball

Ankle sprain is the most frequent of all volleyball injuries. This injury often occurs when a player lands on a teammate's foot after jumping.

A better sense of where your teammates are, stronger ankles, and perhaps high-top shoes can help.

Inexperienced volleyball players are likely to jam their fingers while trying to hit the ball. Should this happen, stop playing and tape or splint the injured fingers.

Bibliography

Cooper, Kenneth. *The New Aerobics*. New York: M. Evans, 1970.

Hollinshead, W. Henry. *Functional Anatomy of the Limbs and Back*. 2d ed. Philadelphia: W. B. Saunders, 1960.

———. *Textbook of Anatomy*. New York: Harper and Row, 1967.

Klafs, C. E., and Arnheim, D. *Modern Principles of Athletic Training*. 4th ed. St. Louis: C. V. Mosby Co., 1977.

Larson, Leonard A. *The Encyclopedia of Sports Medicine*. New York: Macmillan, 1971.

O'Donoghue, D. H. *Treatment of Injuries to Athletes*. 3d ed. Philadelphia: W. B. Saunders, 1976.

Root, L. and Kiernam, T. *The Doctor's Guide to Tennis Elbow, Trick Knee and Other Miseries of the Weekend Athlete*. New York: David McKay and Co., 1974.

Samuels, M., and Wallis, W. *The Well Body Book*. New York: Random House, 1974.

Sheehan, George. *The Encyclopedia of Sports Medicine*. Menlo Park, California: World Publishers, 1972.

Ullyot, Joan. *Women's Running*. Menlo Park, California: World Publishers, 1976.

Wallace, Lynn. *Introduction to Sports Medicine*. 3d ed. Cleveland, Ohio: Case Western Reserve University Press, 1976.

Index

Abrasion, 114
Ankle, 18, 84, 86, 88, 89
Arches, 74, 76, 83
Arthritis, 30, 99
Athlete's foot, 81, 115
Avulsion, 29

Back, 100; injuries, 100–2; pain, 101
Basketball, 76, 88, 93, 98, 110, 117
Bleeding, 23, 24
Blisters, 74, 76, 81, 112–13
Body awareness, 35–37
Bones, 15–16; calcaneus, 81, 85, 90; coccyx, 101, 103; femur, 90, 92, 95, 96, 97, 102; fibula, 86, 88; humerus, 17, 18, 108; iliac crest, 102; knee-cap. See patella; malleolus, lateral, 85, 92; malleolus, medial, 85; meta-tarsals, 81; patella, 96, 98; pelvis, 100, 102; radius, 17, 108; sacrum, 101; scapula, 108; spine, 101; talus, 81, 84, 85; tarsals, 81; tibia, 84, 86, 87, 96, 97; ulna, 19, 108; vertebrae, 100
Bowling, 119
Braces, 78
Brain, 18, 19, 20
Bruise, heel, 84. See Contusion
Bunions, 74, 82

Bursa, 30, 96, 99
Bursitis, 30, 96, 99, 109

Calluses, 114
Cardiopulmonary resuscitation, 24
Cartilage, 17
Cerebral hemispheres, 19
Chafing, 116
Charley horse, 92
Chondromalacia patellae, 99
Contusions, 27, 28, 87, 92
Corns, 74, 114
Cycling, 9, 38, 120–22

Disks, intervertebral, 101; ruptured, 102
Dislocation, 16, 30
Dorsiflexion, 87, 90

Elbow, 16, 17, 18, 107, 109
Endurance, 38
Equipment, 72, 73
Eversion, 87
Exostoses, 81–82
Extension, 18
External otitis. See Swimmer's ear

Fibroblasts, 22
Field hockey, 88, 123, 124

133

Fingers, 18, 110, 117, 119; baseball, 110–11
First aid, 24
Fitness, 38–41
Flat feet. *See* Arches
Flexibility, 42
Flexion, 16; plantar, 86, 90
Foot, 81
Football, 9, 27, 78, 93, 94, 102, 108, 117, 122
Forearm, 16, 17
Fracture, 30–31, 108; stress, 83, 118
Frostbite, 77, 112, 116

Golf, 122
Groin, 103, 104

Hammer toes, 74, 82
Hand, 20, 107
Handball, 21, 123
Heat therapy, 24, 28, 29, 30, 31, 84, 88
Hematoma, 22, 28
Hernia, 103–4
Hip, 18, 92, 96, 100, 102
Hip pointer, 102

Ice, 22, 23
I.C.E., 22, 28, 29, 31, 87, 90, 93, 102
Ice hockey, 102, 123, 124
Ice skating, 103, 124
Inflammation, 22, 29
Inguinal region, 103
Injury repair, 22
Inversion, 87

Jock itch, 112, 115
Jogging. *See* Running
Joints, 16, 27
Jumper's knee. *See* Tendinitis, patellar

Knee, 18, 86, 88, 92, 94–99; water on the, 99

Laceration, 114, 115, 123
Lacrosse, 123
Lateral epicondylitis. *See* Tennis elbow

Lifting, 38, 78
Ligaments, 16, 22, 24, 27, 42, 83, 96; cruciate, 96, 98; deltoid, 85; lateral, 85; lateral collateral, 96; medial collateral, 96, 97, 98; posterior of knee, 96
Lumbosacral pain, 101

Meniscus, lateral, 96; medial, 96, 98
Menstrual problems, 104–5
Minerals, 29, 89, 120
Motor cortex, 19, 20
Muscles, 15, 16, 17, 18, 20, 22, 24, 27, 42; abductors, 18; adductors, 18; antagonists, 18; biceps, 16, 17, 109; cramps, 89; diaphragm, 105; extensors, 18; flexors, 18; gastrocnemius, 47, 90; hamstring, 28, 92, 95; hamstring stretch, 42–45; long peroneal, 92; quadriceps, 29, 92, 95, 98, 99; short peroneal, 92; strain, 28, 29, 76, 93, 108; triceps, 18

Nerves, 18

Orthotics, 76

Pain, 22–23
Patella, 96, 98
Perspiration, 29
Puncture (skin), 114–15

Racketball, 128; injuries. *See also* Tennis
Ringworm, 115
Rugby, 88, 124
Runners, 77, 83, 88, 116
Running, 9, 21, 37, 38, 39, 45, 54, 73, 74, 77, 81, 83, 105, 117, 124

Sciatica, 101
Scrotum, 104
Shin splints, 88
Shoes, 72, 82, 83; fitting, 74; selecting, 73–74
Shoulder, 17, 100, 107, 108; injuries, 108–9; separated, 108
Side ache. *See* Stitch

Skateboards, 126
Skiing: cross-country, 116, 119–20; downhill, 9, 37, 54, 94, 127
Skin, 27, 77, 112
Soccer, 28, 76, 87, 107, 127
Socks, 75, 76
Softball, 110, 114, 128
Sprains, 30, 117; ankle, 85; knee, 97
Squash, 38, 87, 128
Stitch, 105–6
Stretching, 24, 29, 42, 44–50
Sunburn, 112, 116, 120
Surfboard, 128
Surfer's knots, 129
Surfing, 128, 129
Surgery, 30
Swimmer's ear, 129
Swimming, 38, 39, 117, 129
Synovial fluid, 18, 99
Synovial membrane, 17, 96, 108

Tendinitis, 30, 75, 90, 92, 109; patellar, 98, 118
Tendons, 16, 22, 24, 27, 42; Achilles, 90, 92, 118; biceps, 109; injuries to, 89–92; plantaris, 90, 92; rupture, 89, 90; strain, 28, 29, 89
Tennis, 9, 22, 40, 45, 52, 54, 73, 74, 81, 83, 88, 94, 109, 112, 129–30; elbow, 78, 109–10, 123
Tenosynovitis, 30, 90, 109
Throwing, 107, 108, 119, 122, 128
Toenail, ingrown, 82, 83
Toes, 18, 75, 115

Volleyball, 9, 21, 28, 88, 98, 110, 131

Water on the knee: See Knee
Wrist, 18, 107, 110

Yoga, 44